Nutrigenetics

Nutrigenetics

New Concepts for Relieving Hypoglycemia

BY DR. R. O. BRENNAN
with WILLIAM C. MULLIGAN

Foreword by
ROGER J. WILLIAMS, Ph.D.

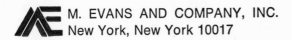
M. EVANS AND COMPANY, INC.
New York, New York 10017

M. Evans and Company titles are distributed in
the United States by the J. B. Lippincott Company,
East Washington Square, Philadelphia, Pa. 19105;
and in Canada by McClelland & Stewart Ltd.,
25 Hollinger Road, Toronto M4B 3G2, Ontario

LIBRARY OF CONGRESS CATALOGING IN PUBLICATION DATA

Brennan, Richard O.
   Nutrigenetics, new concepts for relieving hypoglycemia.

   Includes index.
   1. Hypoglycemia—Nutritional aspects.
I. Mulligan, William C., joint author. II. Title.
RC662.2.B7   616.4′66′0654   75-23063
ISBN 0-87131-187-9

Design by Joel Schick

Manufactured in the United States of America

9 8 7 6 5 4 3 2

Contents

Foreword

Dr. Richard Brennan deserves a tremendous amount of credit for being the founder and god-father of the International Academy of Preventive Medicine. He early saw the vision of a type of medicine which would be concerned with *preventing* disease by cooperating with Nature and using as agents those chemical substances (often nutrients) which are natural constituents of tissue which may be impaired by their lack. He feels very strongly that if we could eat right a tremendous amount of unnecessary disease could be prevented.

He has written this book on hypoglycemia out of his own practical experience. Hypoglycemia is one of the disorders (with a multitude of diverse manifestations) which undoubtedly arises in part from poor and inexpert dietary control. As Dr. Brennan says, the estimates as to the prevalence of this disease vary widely. No one doubts, however, that it afflicts many millions. The imbalance involved can afflict about any tissue or organ and the symptoms, often involving those of a mental character, are liable to be baffling and treated entirely inappropriately unless the nutritional roots are explored.

In Chapter V Dr. Brennan emphasizes the importance of better nutrition education. If nutrition education could be fostered not only in medical schools but also in colleges and universities, high schools and even grade schools, the way would be paved for a far healthier America and the complex problems associated with hypoglycemia would be clarified.

Medical scientists *must* get into the act in a sense not hitherto experienced before the interrelations between disease and nutrition can be brought into scientific perspective.

Dr. Brennan has performed a signal service in medicine and this book about hypoglycemia is an important addition to his contributions.

Roger J. Williams, Ph.D.

Don't Settle for Less-Than-Peak Energy All Day: What Hypoglycemia Is All About

1

In the last century, medical science has made tremendous advances in the diagnosis and treatment of the many ailments and diseases that have plagued mankind; diphtheria, smallpox, typhoid, polio, to name a few, are no longer threatening, and great inroads have been made in the control of diabetes and some forms of cancer. Yet millions of Americans function far below their maximum efficiency, and live from day to day with such problems as dizziness, fatigue, depression, constant anxiety, loss of sex drive, and extreme irritability often verging on violent behavior. Why? First listen to the testimony of two of my patients.

Mr. G: "For the past seven or eight years, I have felt physically sick and mentally confused and depressed. The last three years I have had constant headaches, I've felt tired and exhausted, and hardly had the energy to keep going. It was an effort to make it through the day, after long, sleepless nights.

"During these years, I was going from one doctor to another.

Each would put me in the hospital for several days, and he'd run tests and prescribe various medications for nerves or hormone imbalance. One diagnosed my problem as heart trouble. Then, after thirty days of heart pills, a return to the hospital, and a consultation with two specialists, it was decided it wasn't my heart. Situations like this made me more nervous and apprehensive. I was beginning to doubt my sanity."

And Mrs. B: "For more years than I like to remember, I had suffered from headaches (my main complaint), along with fatigue, insomnia, shortness of breath, spastic stomach, nausea, and anemia.

"I had gone from doctor to doctor, to clinics and to hospitals. Finally, when my temperament deteriorated and when preparing a meal for my family of four became too great a task, I decided I needed a psychiatrist. He told me it was my age (at the time, forty), tension, and nerves. But I had been addicted to sweets since the age of seventeen, and I felt that this had something to do with my condition."

Indeed it did have something to do with Mrs. B.'s condition, as well as Mr. G.'s, and the many Americans with less-than-ideal eating habits who suffer similar symptoms without knowing why and with no one to turn to for help.

These two case histories are representative of hundreds in my files of people who were desperate to the point of giving up and who were tired of repeated visits to doctors who failed to diagnose the root of the problem and, at best, offered only temporary relief. These people were victims of hypoglycemia, a condition in which the body is unable to keep its blood-sugar level up to normal.

The many hypoglycemics who have sought and, fortunately, have found effective treatment are only the tip of the iceberg; scores of men, women, and children in this country suffer, to a greater or lesser degree, from this insidious disorder. And this suffering is completely unnecessary, because hypoglycemia is easily diagnosed by means of a glucose-tolerance test, and can be improved significantly through sound nutrition and proper medical treatment.

I am sure you have experienced, at some time or other, the mid-afternoon "blahs"—that feeling of lethargy and drop in mental alertness that strikes around three or four o'clock and just about finishes you, as far as any real work accomplishments are concerned, for the rest of the day. The self-styled weight watchers who make it a practice to fast for hours during midday and are not as aware as they should be of the body's nutritional needs are especially prone to this syndrome.

Many people accept this drop in energy as a part of their daily routine and regard it as a normal reaction to the stresses and demands of modern living. "Everybody feels that way, so why should I be different?" True, a great percentage of the population is victim to this daily occurrence, caused by a drop in blood-sugar level, but it is *not* normal, and it *can* be eliminated.

Our bodies should have energy to spare all day, from the moment of waking to the moment of falling asleep. This is a feasible goal and one we all should strive for.

The midafternoon fatigue syndrome is the body's cry for help. It is a less severe manifestation of hypoglycemia, but its effects are cumulative and, if left unremedied, will further disturb metabolic balance and cause symptoms like those of the patients quoted above. But even at this point, the situation can be reversed as the power of nutrition works its magic. The dramatic recoveries of these once-troubled people are best appreciated in their own words.

Mr. G. writes: "Within two months of medication and proper nutrition, I was amazed to find myself far more alert, having energy and drive I hadn't experienced in years. My headaches were gone. I couldn't believe it was really me.

"It has now been six months and my overall health is very much improved. I've learned that if I don't eat properly, I begin to feel tired and nervous. My big problem has been changing my eating habits of many years. After eating sweets and sugar-filled foods for so long I'm learning to control myself more each day."

And Mrs. B: "Since changing my eating habits, I feel wonderful. No headaches, chest pains, or stomach trouble. I breathe normally, sleep like I'm getting paid to do so, have more energy than some people who claim to be well, and, of course, my outlook on life has changed for the better."

The return to good health is an indescribable experience, and a change that brings with it an inestimable boost to one's life and career. We never really know how poorly we have been feeling until we encounter in ourselves the vitality and happiness that come only when the body is operating at peak efficiency.

The maxim "You are what you eat" is basically true, and if all of us became more nutrition-wise, much of the ill health in our country would be eliminated. The American way of eating is deplorable, and for that reason both the potential and real menaces of hypoglycemia lurk in everyone. Only you can decide if you wish to follow the dietary habits of the average American, or feel better and stronger every day by providing your body with the correct fuel it needs to function properly.

Know the enemy and what it can do to your system. Hypoglycemia is a condition in which the level of fuel the body needs to function properly is abnormally low during part or most of the day. This fuel is glucose, which the body converts from the sugar in the food we eat. So, when we speak of low blood sugar, a phrase commonly used as a substitute for hypoglycemia, we are actually speaking of a low level of glucose.

When it is well, the body breaks down the carbohydrates found in starches and natural and refined sugars to get the glucose it needs. The glucose it does not immediately need goes to the liver, where it is converted to another form, glycogen, and stored until it is called on. The body's sugar-regulatory system balances the glucose level in the blood to be sure the body is not getting too little or too much. When hypoglycemia attacks, this regulatory system is not working properly.

The immediately apparent answer to the problem would seem to be simply to increase one's intake of sugar or sugar-filled sweets. And that is why the hypoglycemic has a seeming craving for sweets. What his body is really telling him he needs are the vital nutrients it is lacking. The intake of sugar is anything but the right solution, because it has the short-range effect of sharply raising the blood sugar level, causing the body to over-react and sending the blood sugar level to below normal again. This repeated action/reaction process, the long-range effect of sugar intake, causes the body's metabolism to go out of balance. Left unremedied, this imbalance may lead to degenerative disease. Eating sugar to combat hypoglycemia would be like trying to put out a fire with more oxygen.

Researchers know that people who eat a lot of the kind of refined sugar found in such American staples as ice cream, cake, chocolates, and pies are more likely to get hypoglycemia than those who do not eat those products. But sugar is only a single element in hypoglycemia's multiple causes.

Each of us, from the time of conception, is endowed with a unique genetic code. That code determines, in large part, our own particular strengths, weaknesses, and susceptibilities to various disorders. One person may, for example, inherit soft teeth from his or her ancestors, and a resulting severe susceptibiilty to tooth decay. Like other genetic weaknesses, this particular one can be combatted and compensated for with professional care and nutritional supplements.

We all suffer genetic weaknesses, most of which we are unaware of, and we all have differing needs for the various nutritional components that work to compensate for our lacks. Among the possible genetic weaknesses is our own sugar-regulating system. This system is upset not only by nutritional factors, but by genetic factors as well; I call the combined influence of these factors *nutrigenetics*. Hopefully, *nutrigenetics,* as an area of medical study, will someday be recognized. Until science reaches the point of being able to control genetic patterns, we can only offset hereditary weaknesses with good nutrition.

No other illness includes a wider range of problems. When hypoglycemia becomes severe, the immediate effects can be frightening. "I had terrible migraine headaches that lasted several days at a time, as well as allergies and sinus infections that caused my head to feel constantly swollen and sore," an untreated hypoglycemic told me. "I experienced disoriented feelings, dizziness, blurry vision, and feelings of panic. I felt so tired I never wanted to get out of bed. My heart would pound with just the exertion of getting up and my head would feel light and disconnected. "Everything I did required extreme effort. My legs felt like rubber. When I was driving, I would wonder if I could put my foot on the brake. Many times I feared I would pass out because I felt I was in another world. I had constant thoughts of suicide and terrible depressions and crying spells. I had constant diarrhea and my stomach was usually distended and sore."

Any one of more than forty varied and extraordinary symptoms may indicate the presence of hypoglycemia. Dr. Stephen P. Gyland, a Florida physician who himself suffers from the disease, studied more than six hundred hypoglycemic patients and found over seventy percent of them suffering from one or more of these symptoms: nervousness, irritability, exhaustion, faintness (dizziness, tremor, cold sweats, weak spells), depression, vertigo, drowsiness, headaches.

Hypoglycemia is the forerunner of many serious diseases.
Hypoglycemia is a disease in itself, but it can lead to other, more serious diseases if not checked. A person with hypoglycemia also has a concurrently existing problem of *metabolic dysequilibrium,* an imbalance in the chemical processes by which the body feeds and regulates itself. This will have the effect of starving the basic units of life, the cells. When our cells begin to reach a level of starvation, they send out warning signals in the form of the symptoms noted above. And eventually, the repercussions of cell starvation could be felt everywhere, in any body system—nervous, cardiovascular, reproductive, endocrinic (glandular), or digestive.

A good analogy to draw here is with an automobile. A car will not run, of course, without fuel, but driven habitually with a tiny amount or with the wrong kind, it may run well for a while, but eventually every engine component will be adversely affected.

How many Americans have hypoglycemia? No one knows. Estimates begin at ten million. Some investigators believe fifty million would be more accurate. No exact count is available because hypoglycemia is never put on death certificates. People die from more specific chronic, degenerative conditions, such as diabetes or atherosclerosis, the latter a disease that leads to heart attacks or strokes by building soft, fatty deposits in the body's blood vessels until those vessels are too clogged to allow enough blood to flow freely.

As noted, hypoglycemia itself is a chronic, degenerative disease. It is also the forerunner of *all* of the severest forms of the known degenerative diseases. Many researchers speculate that uncontrolled hypoglycemia makes its victims far more susceptible to cardiovascular disease, diabetes, chronic obesity, and even alcoholism.

Cardiovascular or heart disease is the nation's leading cause of death. Though its origins are still unknown, heart disease has been related to hypoglycemia through studies with animals. Each time the test animals' blood-sugar level was lowered, anginal attacks occurred. When a low-carbohydrate, high-protein nutritional program was started, the anginal pains subsided in some animals, and more were relieved when additional nutrients were added by means of various forms of therapeutic augmentation.

Diabetes is our sixth leading cause of death. A remarkable finding is that hypoglycemia always precedes diabetes. Caught in time, hypoglycemia can be treated to prevent most cases of diabetes.

Diabetes is *hyper*glycemia, too *much* sugar or glucose in the blood, and it starts in the same sugar-regulatory system as hypoglycemia. Even the major characteristics of diabetes—excessive appetite, general weakness, itching, constipation, drowsiness, blurred vision, impotence, muscular pains, and neuritis—can be simliar to hypoglycemia's.

It was once thought that the key element in diabetes was that too little of the hormone insulin was produced, that too much glucose, therefore, remained in the bloodstream. Today, investigators know that many diabetic adults produce more than enough insulin to break down or destroy the excess glucose. Like hypoglycemia, then, the causes of diabetes are more complex than first suspected.

Hypoglycemia can provoke symptoms of mental illness. A growing body of evidence also indicates that hypoglycemia may be a *cause* of some mental disorders.

The central nervous system, made up of the brain and spinal cord, supervises and coordinates all body activities. Sensory information is transmitted to the central nervous system, motor impulses pass from it to govern body movements, and it determines much of our behavior. Hypoglycemia deprives this system of the glucose it needs to operate efficiently and may therefore affect behavior adversely.

The central nervous system is the body system most vulnerable to hypoglycemia because it cannot store glucose. It must be fed constantly by the bloodstream, and in situations of acute glucose starvation, it gets first call on available glucose.

Dr. A. Stewart Mason, a British endocrinologist, has reported that hypoglycemia may lead to "emotional outbursts of swearing, shouting or crying associated with slurred speech, staggering gait and a sweat-soaked . . . red face." I have found that people who suffer from schizophrenia or exhibit tendencies toward depression, anxiety, suicide, or generally antisocial behavior frequently have hypoglycemia.

In many of these cases, the hypoglycemic, low-carbohydrate, high-protein nutritional plan leads to remarkable improvement, especially when combined with psychotherapy. But eating the proper foods is not always enough to improve weakened systems. Nutrient augmentation, either orally and/or by injections, under a physician's direction is sometimes necessary.

Some 6½ million Americans are alcoholics. More than 300,000 people will die this year from cirrhosis of the liver, a disease associated with alcoholism. Another 25,000 deaths will occur in automobile accidents caused by drivers influenced by alcohol. Although no one knows how many alcoholics suffer from hypoglycemia, it is known that a substantial number exhibit all the signs of the disease. One of the most telltale characteristics is a craving for sweets. When a person has hypoglycemia, his body tries to compensate by demanding large amounts of sugar, the substance it can most easily and readily turn into glucose. It could be in the form of a piece of chocolate, but it could also be alcohol, which contains sugar and provides the same momentary energy boost.

No one knows how many deaths attributed to alcoholism could be prevented by controlling the alcoholic's hypoglycemic condition. In the few experiments that have been conducted, the hypoglycemic alcoholic was totally freed of addiction with the aid of the hypoglycemic's diet. "I have examined hundreds of patients," reported one psychiatrist, "and found that . . . every alcoholic tested had hypoglycemia."

After many years of treating hypoglycemia, I've found it to be the catalyst in the occurrence of many other physical and mental disorders. These are covered in greater detail in Chapters 8 and 9.

The disease that continues to go undiagnosed. Far more research must be done before hypoglycemia's role in causing serious illness may be understood fully. Yet this research is not being considered by orthodox medicine. Despite hypoglycemia's seriousness, nine out of ten physicians who come in contact with the disease misdiagnose it. "[Hypoglycemia] has remained the stepchild of medicine and is too often not even recognized or then [not] properly treated," writes Dr. Stephen P. Gyland.

The extraordinarily wide range of the symptoms of hypoglycemia allows it to be overlooked or treated *only as a symptom.* The unaware physician, confronted with a wide array of symptoms, can only wonder. Does chronic fatigue indicate anemia? Does vertigo suggest inner-ear trouble? Is the symptom even treatable? The diagnostic trails lead in various directions, usually away from hypoglycemia.

A hypoglycemic does not realize he has low blood sugar. He can only tell the doctor his symptoms and, unless the physician is aware of the disease, he will dismiss his patient as a hypochondriac or continue treating symptom after symptom as each develops. This can be likened to taking an ailing plant and watering, debugging, or repotting it when the real problem is that all it needs is to be fertilized frequently.

Victims of hypoglycemia need help from nutrition-conscious physicians. But only a few of the nation's 114 medical schools have full departments of nutrition. The reason for this lack of attention deals with a medical concept rooted in the nineteenth century. It developed with the discovery of microbes and infectious diseases, when Western medicine devoted itself to the tracking down and elimination of disease microbes, almost to the exclusion of other origins of disease. Two hundred years later, this philosophy still prevails. Yet, at least in the "advanced" nations, it is past time to turn our focus elsewhere. In 1900, more than 600,000 Americans died from infectious diseases. But in 1960, only 50,000 such deaths were reported.

However, the general adult death rate has barely dropped since 1900. The reason: Chronic, *degenerative* diseases are increasing. Cardiovascular disease and cancer alone, for example, account for more than seventy-one percent of the deaths in this country. While orthodox medicine has done a superb job with infectious diseases, it is only now beginning to realize that defeating the microbe is only part of the battle. Much of the balance involves preventive medicine—in large part, good nutrition.

Hypoglycemia or hyperinsulinism? There are three general types of hypoglycemia: a variety that results from a tumor of the pancreas, a type caused by an enlargement of a portion of the pancreas, and the so-called functional hypoglycemia. All but the functional type are rare.

The severity of the pancreas tumor form depends upon the tumor itself—whether it is malignant or benign. If malignant, the cancer will spread and its offshoots will produce insulin throughout the body, creating the terminal condition of uncontrollable low blood sugar. The benign tumor, however, can often be treated dietetically. If diet is unsuccessful, surgical removal of the tumor usually stops the overproduction of insulin.

An enlargement of a collection of cells called the islands of Langerhans, located at one end of the pancreas, is the cause of the second rare form of hypoglycemia. These cells produce all of the body's insulin supply. When the islands expand or become irritated, more insulin is produced. This excess insulin breaks down too much glucose, leaving the body sugar-depleted and suffering from hypoglycemia. This abnormality can be remedied surgically.

Early in the history of hypoglycemia, when its cause was often attributed to tumors or to generalized pancreas enlargement, surgeons were mystified to find neither problem after opening a patient. They then hypothesized that there was a tumor present; they just couldn't find it.

Actually, they were dealing with the third form of the disease, which eventually became known as functional hypoglycemia. Although the chief diagnostician of a leading American clinic claims, "I have never seen a case of functional hypoglycemia," it is the most common variety. It is the type most Americans have.

Because there is no anatomical change in the pancreas in functional hypoglycemia, Dr. Seale Harris, discoverer of functional hypoglycemia, suggested that the drop in blood sugar was in response to a high-carbohydrate diet. He argued that the symptoms could be alleviated by avoiding sugars and starches and by turning to a diet containing more protein.

Functional hypoglycemia originally was called hyperinsulinism. Physicians believed its only cause was the production of too much insulin by the pancreas when the pancreas became overly sensitized to sugar.

Even Dr. Harris made the mistake of assuming hypoglycemia was hyperinsulinism. He found that if less sugar was eaten, less insulin was produced. The blood-sugar level remained steadier. Although he was successful in controlling patients with hyperinsulinism, he did not control completely all hypoglycemics, because only part of their disease was being treated.

It is not unusual in medicine for a single specific condition to be related to a single symptom or to a set of symptoms when a new disease is discovered. As Dr. Harris continued his work and other researchers contributed their own theories, it became evident that low blood sugar was not always caused by overproduction of insulin. Some low blood sugar victims produce normal amounts of insulin. Hyperinsulinism, then, is only one form of the more general disease, hypoglycemia.

Functional hypoglycemia has been further defined recently to include a more subtle form. In this subtle form, called *subclinical hypoglycemia,* symptoms may be vague and diagnosis difficult. A severe hypoglycemic, for example, may have a blood-sugar level that is always below normal. The subclinical victim, however, may show a low level but one still considered normal. It usually does not drop into the hypoglycemic range until the last hours of the prolonged glucose tolerance test.

The dedication of one man. Functional hypoglycemics might still be unrelieved if not for Dr. Harris. A professor of medicine at the University of Alabama in the early 1920s, he took an interest in the work of Dr. Frederick Grant Banting and medical student Charles Herbert Best, the Canadians who discovered insulin's role in diabetes. Diabetes, long a cause of misery and abbreviated life, was presumably controlled after insulin's discovery.

Back in Alabama, however, Dr. Harris's curiosity was aroused when he examined nondiabetic patients who exhibited symptoms of insulin shock, the same insulin shock that diabetics experienced when they took too large a dose of Banting and Best's drug.

When too much insulin is taken, the blood-sugar level drops drastically. Symptoms appear as blood sugar is destroyed too quickly. The patient becomes ravenous. He may faint. Soon his heart begins to beat rapidly. He breaks out into a cold sweat. His vision blurs and his head aches. He begins to tremble as the sudden loss of fuel begins to shut down his body's systems. Delirium and nausea follow. He finally becomes stuporous; his systems have all but stopped in order to conserve what little fuel he has left. He may die if the body does not receive an immediate massive dose of glucose.

The nondiabetic patients who exhibited these symptoms without taking insulin led Dr. Harris to theorize that they were *naturally* secreting too much insulin. He published his theory in 1924 in *The Journal of the American Medical Association*. It was ignored.

Because Banting and Best achieved immediate recognition and Harris did not, because diabetes could be easily diagnosed and hypoglycemia could not, practicing physicians concerned themselves with diabetes while they barely reacted to hypoglycemia. Ennui, when it strikes, strikes at all levels—from the most eminent research laboratories to the smallest private practice.

Banting was cowinner of the 1923 Nobel Prize for physiology

in medicine for his work. Harris continued to gather data, although not many seemed to care.[1]

Dr. Harris meanwhile worked on in relative obscurity. He did not originally name his newfound disease hypoglycemia. He called it "the hunger disease," because of the ravenous appetites of its victims. Also, he discovered a fascinating irony that tied him even closer to Banting and Best during the course of his work in Alabama.

He had borrowed the Canadians' diagnostic test for diabetes, a three-hour examination in which the patient is given 100 milligrams of a sugar solution. The blood-sugar level is then monitored hourly. The patient is considered diabetic if the level exceeds 170 milligrams per 100 cc. of blood. Neither Banting nor Best continued the test past three hours. That was time enough to determine a diabetic condition, they felt. Dr. Harris did extend the test —to six hours—and it is still the best diagnostic test for hypoglycemia.

Dr. Harris also found that some of his patients tended to be both diabetic and hypoglycemic. A similar pattern occurred time after time: A patient would undergo the six-hour glucose test. His level would shoot up beyond normal once the sugar solution, glucose, was administered. Such a patient would have been released and diagnosed as diabetic if the test had been stopped at three hours, but the test continued and the patient's blood sugar plummeted. It would fall so quickly that within two hours it would drop below the diabetic *and* normal range. The patient was, then, hypoglycemic. Harris called this unusual relationship *dysinsulinism*. It is actually diabetes with functional hypoglycemic episodes.

Because of Dr. Harris's work, some physicians, and I am one, believe *all* diabetics are hypoglycemic at one time in their history. We can shrink the mortality rate of diabetes by finding and controlling the early hypoglycemic condition. We *cannot* allow these diseases to attack victims with the answer so near at hand.

---

[1] It took the medical community twenty-five years to recognize Harris's work officially. The AMA awarded him the Distinguished Service Medal in 1949, partially for his research into hypoglycemia. It is the highest award given by the AMA for scientific investigation. Even the citation, however, had little effect in generating interest in hypoglycemia.

Sound nutrition, the foundation of good health. Hypoglycemia exists partially because of an attitude, the attitude that Americans are well nourished. In June 1968, the Department of Health, Education and Welfare (HEW) began its first comprehensive study of malnutrition. Its findings: thirty-five to fifty-five percent of everyone studied in a cross-section of the U.S. population—all income brackets—suffered from one or more nutrient deficiencies.

American children are the hardest hit by malnutrition. One-third of the children studied by HEW had anemia "to a degree that a pediatrician would prescribe therapy right away." In recent years, researchers have found permanent stunting of brain growth and physical growth in babies who suffered from malnutrition before or shortly after birth. The HEW study revealed that fifteen percent of all children it surveyed showed evidence of such growth retardation.

If the suspected millions of hypoglycemic Americans were to eat as well as the man-apes who survived aeons ago on meat and vegetation, most would not have the disease. Diets have been tainted with nutritionally unsound food products.

The worst offender is sugar. Spending fortunes annually through an effective public-relations network and legislative lobby, the sugar industry has convinced most Americans that it is healthful and normal for the average person to eat an average of 104 pounds of refined sugar annually. Sugar provides quick energy and vitality, the industry argues. Sugar processors do not report that sugar is a thief; it has no nutrients, not even the amount necessary for its own absorption by the body's metabolism, a process that must, then, take nutrients from other foods. The body needs no refined sugar. It can convert all the glucose it needs from the starch and protein contained in a high-protein, low-carbohydrate diet and do it more evenly, without the jagged peaks and valleys of glucose excesses and shortages found in the blood-sugar production level of hypoglycemia victims.

The chapters that follow discuss low blood sugar in detail—its complications, diagnosis, and treatment; the serious problem of dietary misconceptions among Americans; and how to guard against or overcome malnutrition with foods high in protein and essential vitamins and minerals. But you may be asking yourself,

What about the ways and means of suddenly reversing one's eating habits of many years? How can this be accomplished without a great deal of difficulty? In the appendix, easily understood tables list the nutrient values of hundreds of the most commonly eaten foods, along with some sample menu plans ranging from 1000 to 2000 calories daily and recipes tied in with those menus. These tables, menus, and recipes will help you make the transition to a genuinely healthy eating regimen as easy and painless as possible.

Three People Whose Lives Were Changed

2

In my twenty-five years of treating hypoglycemia, I've had the good fortune of being able to restore thousands of its distraught victims to good health and happy, constructive lives. These patients' written testimonies, preserved in my files, might seem incredible at first reading, but they represent the truth in every detail and, if anything, understate the startling life changes that recovery from the ravages of metabolic dysequilibrium can bring.

Three representative testimonies appear in the pages that follow. They include case histories of an adult male, an adult female, and a teen-ager and are typical of the many success stories that limitations of space prevent me from including. All names have been changed, but the facts are documented and remain unaltered.

Ralph Miskif was the best salesman for one of the nation's largest producers of business machines. In three years he had doubled his quota, a feat never accomplished by another at the firm. It took him only eight years to work up from a minor sales position in a small business to his present job.

His personnel folder is filled with recommendations for raises and advancement, but the thirty-two-year-old bachelor declined several offers for "management desk duties. He liked active selling." He gloried in being the company's largest source of new business, and his incredible energy enabled him to cover more ground—a sales district encompassing several mid-Atlantic states —than any of his peers.

On a hot summer day three years ago, for the first time in his life, Ralph found his energy flagging. He attributed his fatigue to the stifling weather, although most of his traveling was done in an air-conditioned car. He wanted to be finished with the day's second client so he could go away to relax briefly. He recalled later that it was the first time he "didn't care if he made a sale." The next ninety minutes with his customer passed slowly. Ralph's manner was lackadaisical, abrupt; he paid little attention to the conversation.

His behavior was so unusual that his client, a man he had known since he joined the company, asked if he were sick. He told Ralph he had never seen him so sallow, but the client accepted Ralph's explanation that his strange behavior was due to a recent episode of flu and the warm weather. Ralph *did* get his sale and then excused himself as quickly as he could.

Rather than continue to his next meeting, as he normally would have done, Ralph decided he needed a quick pick-me-up. He stopped at a nearby bar and ordered a double martini. Within minutes, he felt the soothing relief and calming influence of the alcohol. He had three more martinis, called off the remaining two appointments, and returned to his motel to sleep off his drunk.

Ralph's alcoholic binges recurred six times during the next three weeks. On two occasions, he had to call off his appointments, but managed to make his meetings during the other episodes, drinking half a dozen cups of black coffee out of a thermos in an effort to sober up.

The next two months were a nightmare. The constant tension Ralph now found at work was relieved only by pre-lunch and pre-dinner martinis. The more he drank, the less he ate. He always seemed to make it through his morning sales appointments, but by the early afternoon he felt "completely fatigued, as if a plug had been pulled on my energy reserves. I had to have those drinks to keep me going."

His sales fell off sharply. For the first time in seven years and for two consecutive months he was not among the top ten salesmen. Ralph's personality changed so quickly and so drastically that several clients called his employer to ask about his health. His territory was cut so he could have fewer clients, but that didn't solve the problem; it enabled him to drink more and still see his clients.

Ralph talked with his family doctor, who suggested that psychotherapy was the only probable answer.

Two psychiatrists told him that the tension created by his competitive spirit was catching up with him. Both said his drinking was an "escape from reality," nothing more. But Ralph argued that he had always loved competition; he enjoyed winning friends as well as clients. His job was fun before these urges to drink excessively had started. He refused to believe the psychiatrists.

Six months after his initial drinking episode, Ralph's health collapsed and his employers ordered a leave of absence. Ralph then began a quixotic journey to find a physician who could diagnose his problem. Half a dozen doctors gave him a total of more than thirty tests, but none of the tests shed any light.

He was given a prolonged (five-hour) glucose-tolerance test at our clinic because of his symptoms and a family history of diabetes. The test proved Ralph was a severe hypoglycemic.

His diet for the past eight years, high in carbohydrates but low in protein, had created nutritional deficiencies in his body that had finally forced his sugar-regulatory system out of balance. The more carbohydrates he ate or drank, the worse his hypoglycemia became and the further his body's supply of fuel or glucose plummeted. To satisfy his body's ever-increasing demand for energy, he turned unconsciously to the quickest way to get a lot of it— alcohol. In the process, he became an alcoholic.

Ralph had rarely eaten balanced meals because of his constant road trips. For breakfast, he might have orange juice, coffee, waffles drenched in butter and syrup, scrambled eggs, and sausage. Before leaving the motel restaurant, he would fill his coffee thermos and buy candy bars or cookies for a morning break. If convenient, he would stop for a ham sandwich and a beer for lunch. If behind schedule, he had his "portable bar" in the backseat and a can of mixed nuts.

By dinnertime Ralph was starved. As a rule, he dined with a client, and a typical meal might include two double martinis, a steak, a baked potato with butter, cheese, and sour cream topping, avocado-grapefruit salad, seasoned squash, hot rolls, and strawberry shortcake.

He was drinking too much coffee and alcohol while not eating enough protein and vitamin-enriched foods. His daily diet contained close to 5000 calories, a probable excess of 3000 calories a day for his overweight condition. And most of the calories came from carbohydrates and fat.[1]

Ralph received only 460 of those 5000 calories from protein. And he was not receiving nearly enough calcium, phosphorus, vitamins B_1, B_2, D, A, niacin, nor many other nutrients needed by the body.

Once his hypoglycemia was discovered, he was placed on a 2000-calorie, low-carbohydrate, low-fat, and high-protein nutritional plan. He also received therapeutic augmentation of all needed nutrients—vitamins, minerals, amino acids, and unsaturated fatty acids. Now he eats 975 calories daily in protein alone. His glucose level has stabilized and his alcohol problem has diminished because his body no longer craves sugar.

The following two tables break down the nutritional components of Ralph's food intake before and after he was diagnosed

---

[1] Calories are the measurement of the amount of energy-producing value gained from food. Processed and refined carbohydrates are high in energy production but supply *no* vital nutrients (protein, vitamins, minerals, or amino acids) to the body. A diet high in devitalized carbohydrates and low in vital nutrients is therefore a poor one. I use the term *carboholics* to refer to the people who follow this all too familiar eating pattern. The body may use carbohydrates for quick energy, but it cannot use those carbohydrates to build or replenish its tissues and organs, a job that must go on continuously and for which the body must have a steady supply of essential nutrients.

as a hypoglycemic. The first shows his prediagnosis diet and the second the Nutrition-Wise plan that restored him to better health.

FOOD INTAKE BEFORE DIAGNOSIS

4995 Total Daily Calories

CARB.	PROT.	FAT	CA.	PHOS.	IRON	A	B_1	B_2	NIA.	C	D
Cal.			*mg.*		*IU*			*mg.*			*IU*
2675	460	1860	900	1653	25.05	17,087	1.28	2.60	23.50	177	255
(54%)	(9%)	(37%)									

NUTRITION-WISE PLAN

2000 Total Daily Calories

CARB.	PROT.	FAT	CA.	PHOS.	IRON	A	B_1	B_2	NIA.	C	D
Cal.			*mg.*		*IU*			*mg.*			*IU*
645	975	380	1600	3300	25.40	13,632	5.35	24.95	50.45	180	55
(33%)	(49%)	(18%)									

NOTE: See Guide to Abbreviations, APPENDIX I, for all abbreviations used throughout book.

The psychiatrists had been wrong. Ralph went back to work, eating properly, and again began to enjoy his job's competitiveness. Today, two years after his terrifying experience with alcoholism, Ralph is again the number-one salesman in his company.

Mrs. Terri Kanter had not felt well for as long as she could remember. Mother of two elementary-school-age children, she never seemed to build up enough energy during a night's sleep to supply her with the strength she needed to get through the next day. Often she woke in the middle of the night, sometimes because of a nightmare, other times for no apparent reason.

Terri had been married for ten of her thirty-four years, and she loved her husband and enjoyed her children. For the last five years, though, she had slowly grown more irritable, more fatigued, and her problems began to affect her family. There was more bickering with her husband, and her children had come to fear the slightest breach of conduct because of the loud, often painful, retribution it brought from their mother. Terri's husband chastised her on several occasions for being too quick-tempered with them. That, too, led to arguments. She found herself crying more often for reasons she didn't understand.

When the family moved into its new home seven years ago, she took great care in the cleaning and upkeep of the four-bedroom house, but lately she made only halfhearted attempts at housework. She had so little energy that she had to rest between each room. The small garden she had begun had long since given in to weeds but she didn't care. Often the morning dishes went unwashed until late afternoon, and the only reason they were done then was out of fear of her husband's reaction.

"I didn't know there was anything physically wrong with me," she recalled. "I just thought I was naturally hateful or mentally ill and getting worse each year. I yelled at my children constantly and I was always nervous."

In addition to growing fatigue and constant headaches, Terri began having mild fainting spells and blurred vision. When she tried to read herself to sleep at night, she couldn't concentrate on the simplest novel. Her anxiety increased each time she discovered another minor problem developing, and she began to think she was "dying slowly from cancer." It was this thought that finally convinced her to visit a doctor.

As Terri related her complaints and behavior patterns during her first interview with me, her problem became evident. I questioned her about her food habits. She believed they were similar to those of many other women in her age bracket with active families.

She admitted to a constant craving for sweets, and the candy dish and cookie jar were never empty, although she made a large dent in both daily. Her husband was often critical of her having so many sweets in the house, but her reply was, "It's a good way for the kids to get energy." In reality, she ate more candy and cookies than they did.

Terri's diet was incredibly deficient in protein, vitamins, and minerals. For breakfast, she often had only coffee with cream and three teaspoons of sugar. "It's the only way I can get going in the morning, and it's all I have time for," she said.

After the children left for school and her husband for work, she had two additional cups of excessively sweetened coffee and a piece of cake. By noon, her symptoms were severely evident, but she was too busy to care about a good lunch. She knew if the most basic housework wasn't done before midafternoon, she would be too tired to do it at all. Lunch was a cup of tea and cookies. *Terri often ate little protein and had very few necessary nutrients until dinner.*

She thought she could overcome her fatigue during the day by eating so-called high-energy foods. Her favorites were chocolate creams, caramels, and colas, but her subconscious desire for these products was caused solely by her bloodstream's constant low-sugar level.

Terri's hypoglycemic symptoms were at their height when her children completed their after-school play and her hungry husband arrived from work. She hated the evenings, for good reason. It was time for dinner and motherly responsibility, yet it was also the time when she was utterly exhausted. Many of the family's problems started at dinner.

Her poorly balanced meals could easily make hypoglycemics of the rest of the family. She disliked meat, and consequently served small portions of it. Instead, potatoes would abound, along with corn bread. Vegetables might be a can of corn and two sliced tomatoes for the entire family, but for dessert there were often seconds of ice cream and cake.

Terri always went to bed early after a snack of cookies and skim milk. She rarely went out with her husband; she was simply too tired.

Terri literally was suffering from malnutrition. Her poor nutrient intake over the years had thrown her sugar-regulatory system into a state of dysequilibrium. Her body, starved for glucose, was seriously ill, and her sickness stemmed directly from her diet. The Recommended Dietary Allowance (RDA) established by the federal government's Food and Drug Administration for an average adult woman is 2000 calories, 220 of which should come from protein. Terri ate 2500 calories a day, only 150 of them from protein. *Too many of all her daily calories came from carbohydrates.*

She was also deficient in most of the known necessary vitamins and minerals. Her intake of each was far below the RDA and Terri, like others who become ill because of poor eating, needed above-average nutrition if she was to regain her health.

To give her the additional nutrients she needed, her new diet was designed to: reduce her total calories by a quarter; cut her consumption of carbohydrates in half; increase her protein level eight-fold; cut her fat consumption by a third; double her calcium; triple her phosphorus and vitamin C; quadruple her intake of iron and vitamin B_2; increase her vitamin A level six-fold; add fifteen times the amount of thiamine; increase her niacin supply twelve times; and increase her vitamin D consumption eleven times.

Terri's prediagnosis diet is analyzed in the first table that follows and is contrasted with her Nutrition-Wise program as outlined in the second table. Note the large increases in protein and vitamins A and D provided by her Nutrition-Wise plan.

FOOD INTAKE BEFORE DIAGNOSIS

2500 Total Daily Calories

CARB.	PROT.	FAT	CA.	PHOS.	IRON	A	B_1	B_2	NIA.	C	D
Cal.			*mg.*			*IU*			*mg.*		*IU*
1775	150	575	695	805	6.35	2630	0.35	1.15	4.35	62.50	5
(71%)	(6%)	(23%)									

NUTRITION-WISE PLAN

2000 Total Daily Calories

CARB.	PROT.	FAT	CA.	PHOS.	IRON	A	B_1	B_2	NIA.	C	D
Cal.			*mg.*			*IU*			*mg.*		*IU*
640	975	385	1550	3220	25.40	13,682	5.35	5	50.45	180	55
(33%)	(49%)	(18%)									

NOTE: See Guide to Abbreviations, APPENDIX I, for all abbreviations used throughout book.

"It took almost two months before I really began to feel better," Terri told me later. "At first, I would feel well for two or three days and then bad for four or five. But I soon began having more good than bad days, until I was feeling well for months at a time.

"My symptoms now have disappeared. No more crying or depression. No more fatigue or irritability. My husband and I have started what seems like a second honeymoon. Even the children have noticed that I don't yell at them as much. I feel marvelous."

Steve Daniels, seventeen, was suspended from high school in his senior year for three instances of fighting. He was arrested for malicious mischief when he broke the windshield of a car for no apparent reason.

Mr. and Mrs. Daniels had been troubled by their son's misbehavior for three years. "He seemed to be doing so well until then," said Mrs. Daniels. "He received As and Bs as a freshman, was on the student council, and played football or basketball nearly every day."

Steve's teachers that year found him a "natural leader," and his science teacher considered him bright enough to allow him to work on his own rather than on regularly assigned work. For part of the winter, Steve spent his science periods assembling a small computer. Most of his courses were of an advanced level, but Steve's freshman year was his last successful one in high school.

"We didn't know what happened to him," said Mrs. Daniels. "He gradually became more and more sullen and we found him increasingly hard to control. He became careless, then rebellious. We thought at first it was simply a growing stage."

Steve used to come home from basketball or football practice, eat his dinner, and study until he went to bed, but by his junior year, he no longer played any sport and rarely studied. Nothing his parents did seemed to have an effect. They tried to understand, then took a hard line, but neither approach worked.

To school authorities, Steve was no longer leadership material, but a teen-ager who did what he wanted when he wanted. His grades dropped to nearly straight C and he almost failed a history course, not because he wasn't bright, but because he didn't do any work, in class or out. Only his native intelligence kept him in school.

The family doctor found nothing physically wrong with Steve and recommended a psychological evaluation. The psychologist diagnosed Steve as slightly neurotic, but said it wasn't severe enough to cause such a drastic change in his personality. He suggested, however, that Steve begin psychotherapy.

"We really had no choice," Mr. Daniels said. "Steve was on the borderline of delinquency and there were no alternatives."

Psychotherapy failed, and Steve was suspended from school for the third time for fighting. An underclassman had accidentally pushed him in the hall and Steve, in his belligerent attitude, responded by pushing back, harder.

He was told not to return to school. In desperation, his parents took him to several physicians, but none found anything wrong with him. Finally, at our clinic, his glucose level was tested, with the finding that Steve's blood sugar was extremely low. Aware of the tendency of hypoglycemia to worsen toward the end of the afternoon, we discovered that nearly all of Steve's difficulties occurred during the last hour or two of school when his mind became filled with the day's problems and his irritability and temper increased.

Mrs. Daniels accused herself when the diagnosis was made; she allowed Steve his extra twenty minutes of sleep in the morning because he was constantly tired. This gave him only enough time for his customary glass of juice and two doughnuts.

"He wouldn't even let me pack him a lunch," Mrs. Daniels said. "So I don't know what he ate during the day." What Steve ate was whatever he could get from vending machines, and this was usually the sweet candy products that made him feel better. And sometimes after school he went to a local coffee shop where he usually had a hamburger along with two colas and an ice cream cone.

His poor eating continued at the dinner table. Mrs. Daniels suspected that Steve ate little during the day, so she tried to give him the food he liked, dishes rich with cream sauces and extra desserts.

Steve immediately was put on a low-carbohydrate, high-protein diet, consisting of half as many carbohydrates as before, but three times as much protein. In addition, he received large dosages of needed nutrients in capsule form.

Steve's before-and-after food intake is compared in the following two tables.

FOOD INTAKE BEFORE DIAGNOSIS

3760 Total Daily Calories

CARB.	PROT.	FAT	CA.	PHOS.	IRON	A	B₁	B₂	NIA.	C	D
	Cal.			*mg.*		*IU*			*mg.*		*IU*
2295	548	917	795	1683	19.30	3685	1.35	1.50	12,380	221	105
(61%)	(15%)	(24%)									

NUTRITION-WISE PLAN

2000 Total Daily Calories

CARB.	PROT.	FAT	CA.	PHOS.	IRON	A	B₁	B₂	NIA.	C	D
	Cal.			*mg.*		*IU*			*mg.*		*IU*
650	985	385	1600	3300	25.40	13,682	5.35	24.95	50.45	180	60
(33%)	(49%)	(18%)									

NOTE: See Guide to Abbreviations, APPENDIX I, for all abbreviations used throughout book.

Steve's symptoms disappeared within three months, but it was too late to correct the damage he had done to his academic future. In ninth grade he had dreamed of acceptance to an Ivy League school, but his high-school record precluded that chance. Instead, he entered a junior college where he was named to the dean's list all four semesters. He was recently accepted by a large west-coast university.

Nutrigenetics: How Malnutrition and Genetic Weaknesses Cause Hypoglycemia

3

German pathologist Rudolf von Virchow said in 1858: "The body is a cell state in which every cell is a citizen." The body contains about one quadrillion cells. Each has its own job and, like any good citizen, each must be in good health to do it properly.

Orthodox medicine finds it difficult to accept the premise that disease can originate because of a cellular imbalance. Yet the cell represents the total organism's health. It is the base from which the body's tissues, organs, and systems pyramid.

Two factors that create a metabolic imbalance within the cell: malnutrition and genetic weakness. Malnutrition can affect metabolic balance, because the bloodstream can only supply the cells with what it draws from food. When this food is lacking in vital nutrients, functions within the cell are impaired. In addition, metabolic imbalances evolve more easily when there is a weakness in the "genetic blueprint," the hereditary factors carried by our genes.

Thus, metabolic inequities and the degenerative diseases they lead to strike when these two factors occur simultaneously. Functional hypoglycemia, for example, is caused when an individual who suffers from a specific genetic weakness fails to strengthen it with nutritious eating. The cause then is *nutrigenetic*, a combined form of nutritive and genetic influences.

The uncorrected nutrigenetic factor creates a chemical imbalance called metabolic dysequilibrium. Hypoglycemia is exactly that—an imbalance in the sugar-regulatory system that prevents the maintenance of a stable blood-sugar level.

The degree of the imbalance determines the degree of the illness. Death occurs when balance is lost completely.

The cell is always affected first. It does not live alone, however, but with its quadrillion neighbors. Groups of them combine to form tissues, glands, and organs. When the cell loses its efficiency, so do the larger cellular communities. The entire body suffers.

The incidence of hypoglycemia and other chronic, degenerative diseases is increasing. Genetic changes take time to develop and cannot alone explain the extraordinary rise in chronic diseases. This means that more Americans are not eating well. When an individual is malnourished for an extended period, his body loses the ability to hide its genetic weaknesses (which everyone has to some degree and which are difficult to determine). The result is that his body chemistry becomes imbalanced. But the body can support its weak spots when it is nourished properly. This is because genes are not the fleshed-out pattern of the body's biochemical life, only the blueprint. Anyone can complete the design, buttressing weak spots, by eating according to his own needs. But hypoglycemics must eat more nutritiously to reestablish a chemical balance that has been lost for some time.

Each individual's needs are unique. No one nutritional program will supply everyone with the exact nutrients he needs; no average man or woman exists. Everyone has different-sized organs, which function more or less efficiently. Some are more susceptible to disease, others more resistant. Some need less of a certain nutrient, others more.

"In no other species are the differences between individuals so great as the human race, . . ." Julian Huxley wrote in *Psychology Today*. No two people in the world have the same hereditary characteristics carried in the body's estimated 100,000 genes.

Dr. Linus Pauling points out that if there were only five hundred genes in the human body, there would be only a ten percent chance that one person would fit the exact "normal" pattern for all traits. Nutritious eating, however, benefits everyone. The closer an individual gets to eating what is, for him, a perfect diet, the better he will feel.

Unfortunately, no one lives on a perfect diet. Man did not know what a good diet was for most of history. Today he is closer to that understanding, but he is still affected by poor eating conditions of the past. The inferior diets of former generations have left their mark on him.

These deficiencies will continue to haunt future generations. The longer man takes to reach an optimum diet, the longer he will take to reach optimum health. "The change that might be brought about by the adoption of a scientific diet would be a very spectacular and decided change," Dr. D. T. Quigley wrote in 1943. "Somewhere from 70 to 80 percent of the disease that now afflicts the human animal *would be eliminated* [emphasis added]. The average age . . . could be extended . . . to well over one hundred years. No one has yet known what the upper age limit could be under optimum conditions. . . . The life period may be doubled."

The body must have thousands of different products in proper proportions to reach near-perfect health. Many of these products are made in the body from a smaller group of raw materials: vitamins, minerals, carbohydrates, fats, proteins, and, of course, water. The proportions differ with the individual.

To eat these items in the right quantities, however, does not guarantee health, which depends also on the body's reaction to these nutrients and its use of them. The cell will still lack fuel if the nutrients are improperly digested or assimilated.

All bodily systems are "go" when perfect balance exists.
A system of arteries, veins, and capillaries—"pipes" that differ in size—transport fuel throughout the body. Arteries are the conduits

for "unused" blood that provides the body's tissues with oxygen, glucose, and nutrients. Veins carry away "used" blood and the waste products produced by the cells. The capillaries are minute conduits through which oxygen is released to the tissues.

These vessels may be affected by nutrigenetic disease, because each blood vessel is composed of living cells that need their own supply of nutrients to function. The genetic blueprint can make an individual's arteries and veins more susceptible to disease, while a poor diet almost assures it.

The stomach and intestines, with help from the pancreas and liver, digest and absorb food. Food is broken down into simple compounds in the stomach and intestines where enzymes and other digestive juices interact. The body absorbs these products through the intestine. But a disease cycle can develop in these systems also. The result is the same as if there were a breakdown in a transport system: Nutrients fail to reach the cell and the effect is cumulatively degenerative.

The components of the sugar-regulatory system, beyond the cellular level, are the autonomic nervous system, the endocrine system, and the liver.

The *autonomic nervous system* controls the involuntary and unconscious activity of the body: for example, the heartbeat, the stomach's digestive action, the contractions of the intestine, and the bladder's excretory activity.

The *endocrine system* comprises a group of glands that secrete their fluids (hormones) directly into the bloodstream rather than through a duct to a specific area. By passing their secretions into the blood, their effects are felt throughout the body. These glands secrete twenty-eight known hormones, which regulate all body activities. Three glands especially affect the blood-sugar level: the pancreas, the adrenals, and the pituitary.

The pancreas is both an endocrine and an exocrine gland (an exocrine gland is one that has a duct and therefore delivers its hormone directly to a specific area). The duct of the pancreas delivers pancreatic juice into the small intestines to aid digestion. The endocrine function involves glucose regulation.

The pancreas secretes two endocrine hormones from the islands of Langerhans, the cluster of mazelike cells at the gland's base. Two types of cells there produce insulin and glucagon.

Beta cells produce insulin, the hormone capable of lowering blood sugar. Insulin accomplishes this purpose in several ways: It stimulates the liver to remove sugar from the bloodstream and store it as glycogen; it inhibits the liver from releasing any of its stored sugar supply back into the bloodstream; it stimulates muscles to burn glucose at a higher rate; it acts as a catalyst to enable cells to draw and absorb glucose from the blood.

The alpha cells of the islands of Langerhans produce glucagon, which can force the liver to release its stored sugar into the bloodstream. Glucagon counteracts insulin and plays a necessary role in maintaining the endocrine system's balance.

The second of the endocrine system's triumvirate of sugar-regulating glands are the adrenals. These glands also produce two major hormones, adrenalin and glucocorticoid, both of which help maintain the blood-sugar level. Adrenalin stimulates the liver to change glycogen back to glucose, just as glucagon does. Adrenalin, however, is secreted only in times of crisis. It gives the body more fuel to fight or run and raises the heartbeat and blood pressure to move the additional fuel through the body. Glucocorticoid, which also reconverts glycogen to glucose, is released during normal body activity.

The pituitary gland is located at the base of the brain. Although no bigger than a large pea, it's the endocrine system's command gland, and it takes orders directly from the brain. The multipurpose pituitary is deeply involved in blood-sugar regulation. It tells the adrenals when to ask for more insulin, it forces the pancreas to produce insulin when too much glucose appears in the blood, and it also produces growth hormones, which tend to lower blood-sugar levels.

The *liver*, the third component of the sugar-regulatory system, is one of the largest organs in the body. It has an estimated one hundred functions to perform in addition to storing glycogen. It can release glycogen and absorb glucose at the same time because it possesses a double blood supply. The liver's importance is great: One-quarter of the body's entire blood supply must pass through it every minute.

All parts of the regulatory system must be perfectly in balance if the body is to remain healthy. Each must know exactly what the other is doing.

The liver and endocrine system monitor each other through the central nervous system. The brain's hypothalamus is partially responsible for the sugar-regulatory system: It watches over the autonomic nervous system; it directs the pituitary; it monitors the liver. The brain assures the complete interdependency of each of these systems with the normal function of the body.

How does the body's sugar-regulatory system work? Much of the food we eat is absorbed from the intestinal tract and sent into the bloodstream in the form of glucose, so blood-sugar concentration increases. The increase activates the pancreas to produce insulin. The liver is then stimulated to withdraw glucose from the blood passing through it and store it as glycogen. The liver will not release any glycogen because of the high level of insulin still in the bloodstream.

Once the food is absorbed completely, the insulin rate lowers, as there is less glucose in the blood. When the blood sugar drops below a certain level several hours after the food has been absorbed, the liver will begin to reconvert its stored glycogen back to glucose and return it to the bloodstream at a rate sufficient to serve tissue needs.

If food is withheld or the blood-sugar level falls below bodily demand, hormones from the pituitary and pancreas are called upon by the hypothalamus. Glucagon is released as an added stimulant to increase the flow of glucose from the liver. The liver will continue to turn glycogen into glucose as long as it is stimulated. When the liver runs out of glycogen, the pituitary hormone, ACTH, causes fat in the form of fatty acids to enter the bloodstream from its storage areas around the body.[1] But the liver's production of glucose from products other than glycogen is less efficient. The body will soon react to this increased load with symptoms of fatigue and nausea.

---

[1] The liver can take fatty acids, as well as starch and protein, and convert them to glucose.

The blood-sugar level should remain between 80 and 120 milligrams per 100 cc of blood when fasting. At lower levels, an individual is normally hungry. It should not jump more than 70 milligrams after a meal or drop below 80 milligrams after several hours of fasting. When it does, it means that one or more of the opposing factors in the sugar-regulatory mechanism is disturbed and the proper balance destroyed. The result is diabetes or hypoglycemia, or both. Diabetes is a label for extraordinarily high levels, while hypoglycemia is the medical name for the cause of low or unstable levels.

Disease-triggering factors. Many people may continue functioning for a long time with the nutrigenetic factor present without getting hypoglycemia. Eventually, one of many factors will trigger the disease. Here is just a partial list of possible catalysts:

I. *Inadequate nutrition because of*
    poverty
    improper preparation of food
    lack of availability of food
    cultural patterns
    dieting for weight loss
    chronic alcoholism
    advanced age
    restricted diets for other diseases
    psychiatric disorders
    pregnancy

II. *Impaired absorption because of*
    gastrointestinal disturbances (chronic diarrhea, colitis, coeliac disease, tuberculosis, absence of bile, surgical resection of the intestinal tract, persistent vomiting as in pregnancy or chronic intestinal obstruction, dysentery, cystic fibrosis of the pancreas)
    excessive use of mineral oil
    cardiovascular disease
    advanced age

III. *Inadequate use or storage because of*
    diabetes mellitus

advanced disease of kidney, liver, or pancreas
hypothyroidism
antibiotic therapy
malignancy

IV. *Increased body requirements because of*
hyperthyroidism
fever
physical exertion
pregnancy
lactation
environmental extremes
rapid growth
postsurgical procedures
injuries
certain toxic agents
burns
convalescence
infections
stress

These triggers, however, will be less likely to initiate hypoglycemia, even with the hereditary factor present, if a high-protein, low-carbohydrate diet is being followed.

A poor diet affects all of the sugar-regulatory system's parts. The endocrine system, for example, gets its supply of hormone-producing material from food. If the pancreas isn't given enough nutrient, too little insulin may be produced, because it can be made only from what the body absorbs. Too little insulin will create a diabetic condition. The same is true if a poor diet affects the alpha cells in the islands of Langerhans. The result would be too little glycogen being converted, and, thus, hypoglycemia.

A diet high in carbohydrates, especially sugar, and low in protein is the diet that most often leads to hypoglycemia. Dr. A. M. Cohen of Israel has shown that sugar-fed rats develop abnormalities in the islands of Langerhans. Dr. John Yudkin of England has discovered that rats also develop enlarged adrenal glands from a high-sugar diet. By decreasing the amount of sugar in the diet, the severe jumps and drops of diabetics and hypoglycemics tend to become more even. The steadier the blood-glucose level, the healthier the individual.

University of Michigan medical school investigators Jerome W. Conn and L. H. Newburgh found that sugar levels were most balanced when blood sugar was produced from protein, not from refined carbohydrates. Protein takes longer to be digested, absorbed, and metabolized in the blood. U.S. Department of Agriculture researchers suggest that, because protein does take longer, the bloodstream receives a steadier supply of glucose.

If Americans were getting enough protein and other nutrients, eating sugar (which lacks nutrients), would not cause as much damage as it does. A Mysore, India, experiment showed that the sugar level remained relatively healthy and steady when glucose was eaten with high amounts of protein. Only alone, in snacks and desserts, do carbohydrates cause the large peaks and valleys in the blood-sugar level.

The effect of a diet rich in these empty calories is comparable to the effect produced by the degeneration of batteries in a flashlight. The beam is bright when the batteries are new. Week by week, the beam dims, whether or not the flashlight is used, until only a glimmer remains. The stored energy in the battery has been dissipated. The same result occurs with the average American diet. To recharge the body's dissipated energy, however, takes a lot more time and a lot more money than it does to replace flashlight batteries.

Sugar and Refined Flour:
Public Enemies Number
One and Two

4

Man's attraction to sweetness began thousands of years ago when his forerunners discovered bee's honey and wild fruit. But nomadic man continued to forage for sweet delicacies for centuries without discovering a way to keep them near. About 550 B.C., however, after man had learned to farm, an unknown but farsighted experimenter in the northeastern area of what is now India found that, by extracting and drying the fluid of a certain plant, he could produce a similar sweetness without having to fend off a bee's swarm. The plant was sugarcane and the fluid, or sap, sucrose.

Sugarcane was cultivated only in that area of India for a thousand years until traders took it west to Egypt and east to China. It followed the expansion of the known world to Africa and the Mideast. It went with the Spanish explorers to Brazil and the Caribbean, and Christopher Columbus planted the first cane stalks in the West Indies in 1494.

Sugar remained a luxury even with the discovery of tropical areas in which sugarcane could grow. It remained a nobleman's food well into the eighteenth century when Caribbean markets and slave labor sent the cost spiraling downward. The masses took sugar to heart only around 1750, when the refining process began to develop rapidly. And except for brief periods during wars, world sugar consumption has continued to rise at an astounding rate.

While refined-sugar consumption mushroomed, a corresponding decrease occurred in other carbohydrates, the complex sugars such as the starches found in potatoes and rice. The complex sugars are infinitely better for the body's sugar-regulatory system because they contain nutrients and are less likely to cause the severe metabolic imbalance of the sugar system that sucrose does.

Sugar consumption continues to rise. World consumption of sugar has increased faster than that of any other food, by a hundred percent between 1938 and 1958 according to a report by the United Nations Food and Agriculture Organization (FAO). The FAO's study, concluded in 1958, is the latest worldwide sugar report available. Although dated, it nevertheless shows sugar's incredible international popularity since World War II.

Dr. John Yudkin, a British physician and biochemist who has studied sugar's effects on humans and animals for more than twenty-five years, found in 1958 that 650 million people in nine underdeveloped nations ate 105 percent more sugar than they did prior to World War II. These people ate nine percent less meat and seven percent less protein. They were getting more calories, but calories devoid of essential vitamins, minerals, fats, and amino acids. Dr. Yudkin reported that a quarter of the world's population ate better before World War II than it did in 1954. It was the quarter with the lowest rate of food consumption, the one that most needed the more nutritious foods. Instead, the sugar consumption rate rose and rises still.

The population of the United States consumes over 100 pounds of sugar per person annually, second only to England. That figure is approximately one-sixth of the population's total diet. The world's population ate only three pounds of sugar per person annually just 150 years ago.

Sugar eating increases with a nation's wealth up to a point. The

United States and Great Britain have long been leaders in sugar consumption, but within the last ten years their rates have stabilized. It is the newly rich or growing nations that now have the largest growth.

Sugar is a metabolic thief. The increase in sugar consumption is often at the expense of other necessary foods, with a corresponding loss in nutrient values. Refined sugar contains nothing but carbohydrate calories, but even the raw, unprocessed product contains only one half of one percent of the minimum daily requirements of vitamin B_1, one percent of B_2, two percent of calcium, and five percent of iron.

Sugar does not contain the ingredients needed for its own metabolism by the body as most nutritious foods do. Consequently, the nutrients needed to break down pure cane sugar must be robbed from other foods, causing them to become deficient, or it must be taken from the body's tissues. But the tissues of millions of people are already deficient because of malnutrition. Their bodies limp along, depleted, with their reserves constantly being siphoned. And with reserves already inadequate, disease is sure to strike. Thus, sugar is not only composed of empty calories, devoid of any nutritional value, but is composed of sickness-breeding calories, "malignant" calories that actually destroy health.

If sugar lacks all vital nutrients, if the body can maintain its glucose fuel supply without it, why is sugar eaten?

No physiological reasons are known, but people may become psychologically dependent on carbohydrates, especially if their childhood diets were high in them. These individuals receive many calories, which fatten them, but they remain poorly nourished. This is why nutritionists object to obesity being called "overnutrition." Sugar, more than other food, can cause obesity while producing malnutrition.

The sugar industry and misleading promotion. Sugar's supposed benefits are constantly brought to the public's attention through the sugar industry's lobbying agencies such as Sugar Information, Inc. One of this agency's favorite ploys is to suggest that sugar is a necessary element in body metabolism: "the fuel of life." It should be called the "fool's nectar."

Such a statement is misleading; it deliberately confuses sucrose with glucose. The sugar industry knows that *cane sugar* and *blood sugar* are two different compounds entirely.

Claims of increased energy by sugar-industry advertisements were recently challenged by the Federal Trade Commission. The commission objected to what it called "deceptive" advertising. The Amstar Corporation, which owns Domino sugar, agreed to conform to an FTC demand to advertise a corrected statement in one of every four of its ads for one year. The statement clarifies the company's representation of the product as a source of "strength, energy and stamina." Part of the correction says ". . . Actually, Domino is not a special or unique source of strength, energy and stamina. No sugar is, because what you need is a balanced diet and plenty of rest and exercise."

The National Advertising Review Board forced the Sugar Association to promise in February 1973 not to use an advertising claim that noted: "Sugar. It isn't just good flavor, it's good food."

The Sugar Association agreed to withdraw the claim until it said it could prove the statement true. At this writing, no proof has been provided.

The five-member panel of the National Advertising Review Board also took umbrage at the Sugar Association's ad titled, "The Sweet Side of Good Nutrition," which included in its copy the statement: "Sugar isn't the only nutrient in an ice cream cone." The panel suggested the sentence was "inaccurate and misleading because it implied that sugar is a nutrient."

These incidents are two of the few that puncture the myth the sugar industry so diligently cultivates.

Sugar or cyclamates—which is the least harmful? The sugar industry also uses its vast advertising campaigns to protect its interests. One of its most successful efforts was the purge of cyclamates from American markets. Cyclamate, of course, was the non-sugar-sweetening additive that conserved calories for dieters and diabetics. Cyclamates were widely distributed for ten years, but on February 14, 1970, all were ordered off the market by the Food and Drug Administration because of reports that the sweetener caused bladder cancer, birth defects, and animal mutations.

Much of this research was initiated and compiled by the sugar industry, which then popularized these studies with extensive advertising. As early as 1957, the industry spent $750,000 on the testing of cyclamate. It then took its argument to the government and the people. "Sugar's got what it takes," read one advertisement. "It's instant energy. Soft drinks made with sugar give you something to go on. But 'syntha-colas' made with chemicals only give a wet, sweet taste."

The evidence mounted. Abbott Laboratories, the largest producer of cyclamate, plied its test rats with massive quantities of the chemical, the equivalent in man of eleven pounds of cyclamate a day for two years. Initial evidence led to the sensationalized headlines of 1969/1970 that labeled cyclamate a "health hazard" or a "producer of bladder cancer." The rats actually developed the first signs of a bladder cancer only after eating huge amounts.

Cyclamates had become a threat to the sugar industry, and the industry retaliated. Now that the backlash has receded and the industry's paranoia subsided, Abbott Laboratories is quietly attempting to reverse the FDA's 1969 decision. Abbott claims new studies show cyclamates are harmless, at least less harmful than sugar.

Abbott gained strong support from *Medical Tribune,* a medical newspaper and the British journal, *Nature,* if only indirectly, when both published vitriolic editorials on the sugar industry and its part in the cyclamate ban.

Nature wondered whether "scientific advisers or the politicians who manipulated them look the more ridiculous." It also called evidence that cyclamates are potential carcinogens "about as solid as candy floss."

Medical Tribune was more specific:

"Throughout . . . there were other nasty rumors to the effect that the publicity and pressure for removal of the cyclamates was a result of activities of 'the sugar lobby.' More recently, a study in West Germany on 832 rats receiving cyclamates revealed bladder cancer in only one, and that was unrelated to dosage. The investigator concluded that the tumor was unrelated to cyclamates. . . . Malignancies in man have yet to be linked to cyclamates."

The newspaper also noted that Nobel Prize recipient Denis P. Burkitt "observed in man that . . . intestinal malignancies and other intestinal disorders were related to diets high in refined carbohydrates."

Now that more people are becoming aware of sugar's dangers, the sugar industry is planting the roots of its latest myth: Brown sugar is better than white. Little difference exists between white and brown sugar except in the degree of refinement. Brown sugar has no nutrients either. The process in both cases makes the finished product absolutely pure: Neither impurities nor nutrients remain.

Noncaloric sweeteners, although artificial and nonnutritive, are far less dangerous than sugar. These products can be used as sugar substitutes but should not be relied on permanently. Once you are eating nutritionally, the desire for sweetening will lessen naturally.

Many ailments are directly related to sugar. There is evidence that sugar may cause harm to the skin, eyes, liver, and hormones. Its use is related to gout, some forms of cancer, and diverticulitis (an intestinal disorder) in test animals. Research physician Dr. D. T. Quigley, as early as 1943, said: ". . . Every ounce of sugar that is taken into the human economy reduces the ability to resist infection, as it furnishes only calories and none of the elements which protect against infections. . . ."

Dr. Yudkin found that patients suffering from a skin disease called seborrheic dermatitis, which causes the skin's glands to oversecrete an oily substance, ate substantially more sugar than those without the skin disease. Bottle-fed babies who have sucrose in their formulas rather than the mother's natural sugar (lactose) often have stomach ailments. Sugar consumption tends to fatten the liver and make it produce more enzymes, which can throw the body's cholesterol production out of kilter. (Cholesterol is part of the material that forms in the arteries, causing atherosclerosis.)

A 1964 Japanese study reported that coffee—its caffeine—and sugar consumption often are related to cancer of the urogenital and digestive organs. Prostate cancers were especially significant. Higher rates of breast, ovarian, bladder, intestinal, and rectal cancers also were found in high-quantity sugar consumers. Five American researchers reported that increased blood-sugar levels corresponded with cervical cancer.

Gout, too, may be triggered by eating large amounts of sugar. Gout attacks nearly any joint in the body, although the classical attack is of the large toe. Many cases not connected with the feet are thus mistaken for bursitis or arthritis, but the disease is not as rare as believed by many physicians. Here, too, an inherited characteristic is thought to be part of the cause. The genetic trait causes the abnormal metabolism of certain compounds in the body called purines, which are then not broken down properly; a residue is left, uric acid. The uric acid may build up in joints sufficiently to cause the swelling and pain of gout. Patients with this problem studied by Dr. Yudkin were found to be eating nearly twice as much sugar as the control group.

Here again is the nutrigenetic factor—the inherited genetic deficiency coupled with malnutrition. The gout victim's genetic weakness is enhanced and allowed to surface because he does not protect himself with good nutrition. Of course, in some cases, the weakness may be so intense that nothing will prevent it. But these are exceptions, not the rule.

Several researchers have discovered that microbes in the colon that help in digestion differ in type and number between large-quantity sugar consumers and those who are not. The differences are enough to affect the function of the colon and enough to cause diverticulitis, which causes severe pain and diarrhea in the large intestine.

Several animal studies in which a high-quantity sugar regime was followed shortened the life-span of rats. If these early experiments prove valid for humans, many large-quantity consumers of sugar products may be eating as much as ten years off their lives.

Sugar was earlier defined as a metabolic thief, harmful to good health. In this sense, it is no better than the illegal hard drugs that satisfy the addict's craving for a physical pleasure but do not satisfy any of his nutritional needs. Sugar, like heroin, should be banned. I hope we will soon see the day when sugar will be labeled "CAUTION. MAY BE DANGEROUS TO YOUR HEALTH."

Refined flour: enemy number two. The grains that compose our processed white flour and breads are more of the malignant calories Americans eat that contribute to malnutrition. These are not *naturally* empty; man has made them so.

The industrial age of the late eighteenth century changed the milling process of grains. Grains were once prepared for cooking by being ground in a stone mill, and as much as eighty-five percent of the whole grain remained in the flour with this method.

The advent of the industrial age and a growing population with an increased demand for bread and mercantile pressures brought the rolling mill. The new mill could produce much more flour than the stone mill, but unfortunately it generated enough heat to destroy most of the grain's protein along with wheat germ and its oil. It removed the outer coating of the grain as well as its hull and, in so doing, removed most of the nutrients and bulk we need.

The flour was bleached, aged, and preserved, usually with chlorine dioxide. This chemical further destroyed many essential oils and amino acids.

What was left was the grain's starch. The new process made grain much like sugar, full of quick, short-lived energy, but lacking constructive, long-term power. There was immediate "gas for the engine," but not enough to maintain the body parts needed to use the fuel efficiently.

Processed flour was perfect for merchants. It kept much longer than its stone-ground counterpart (which lasts no more than three weeks). Insects were not attracted to it (there are not enough nutrients in it to keep them alive) and, because production increased, stores had more to sell.

The fact that seventy-five percent of the value of the natural whole grain was extracted concerned relatively few.

Today's white bread, hardly the "staff of life." The following table lists the natural nutrients that exist in wheat grain, the percentage of each removed in the production of white bread, and the known, and possible, biological complications that may occur in humans when a deficiency arises in any one of these nutrients:

NUTRIENT	PERCENTAGE REMOVED	DEFICIENCY EFFECT
Vitamin A	90	Poor vision; possible influence on arthritis and reproductive failure.
Vitamin B$_1$	77	Derangement of appetite control; beriberi; possible influence on mental illness, heart damage, and mental retardation.
Vitamin B$_2$	80	Possible influence on congenital defects, rheumatoid arthritis, and mucous membrane difficulties.
Vitamin B$_3$	81	Pellagra; possible influence on mental illness and rheumatoid arthritis.
Vitamin B$_6$	72	Possible inefficiency in using amino acids; possible influence on convulsive seizures, arthritis, and mental illness.
Vitamin B$_{12}$	77	Influence on genetic damage.
Pantothenic Acid	50	Inability to produce steroid hormones; possible influence on infertility, congenital defects, and mental disease.
Vitamin D	90	Difficulty in using calcium and phosphorus.
Vitamin E	86	Weakness in cell membranes; possible influence on heart disease and aging.
Folic Acid	67	Possible genetic damage; congenital defects; infertility; mental illness; some cancers and heart disease.

NUTRIENT	PERCENTAGE REMOVED	DEFICIENCY EFFECT
Calcium	60	Poor bone formation; possible influence on infertility.
Chromium	40	Influence on heart disease and diabetes.
Cobalt	89	Poor red blood cell development; possible influence on sterility.
Iron	76	Anemia; possible influence in obstetrical complications.
Magnesium	85	Improper energy exchange within cell; possible influence on alcoholism, mental illness, and heart disease.
Manganese	86	Possible influence on sterility and mental illness.
Phosphorus	71	Improper energy exchange throughout body; possible influence on congenital defects and infertility.
Potassium	77	Imbalance in cellular fluid regulation; possible influence on mental illness.
Selenium	16	Liver deterioration.
Sodium	78	Imbalance of body fluids; possible influence on infertility.
Choline	30	Instability of cell membrane; possible influence in some cancers and heart disease.
Zinc	78	Possible influence on congenital deficiencies, infertility.

"Enrichment"—a feeble gesture. The flour industry did nothing to improve its product until it was pressured to do so in 1941. The resulting "enrichment," however, meant replacement of thiamine (vitamin B_1), riboflavin (B_2), niacin (B_3), and iron. *That was all*. Processing took out parts of twenty-two elements. The industry put back parts of four.

The flour industry has not bothered to add another nutrient in over thirty years, in spite of continued research that has revealed many additional bodily needs from grain's natural ingredients. In fact, sixty percent *less* vitamin fortification is added to flour today than was twenty years ago. The food is still deficient. Yet the bakers of white bread are allowed to print the word "enriched" on their labels. Nutritionist Roger J. Williams notes that rats given a diet of this "enriched" bread either died or became stunted.

The Food and Drug Administration finally ordered bakeries to double white bread's iron content to reduce iron-deficiency anemia, a fast-growing problem among Americans. The addition of only one of the nutrients lost in the processing of white flour, or even the addition of ten, will not compensate for the loss of the complete food that natural wheat grain is. Even so, the FDA's order met stiff opposition from many doctors who feared that too much iron would be ingested causing physiological problems such as kidney failure and heart disease. This reaction prompted the FDA to countermand its order for greater iron content.

Whole-grain bread, yes; white bread, no. Unlike white and brown sugar, there is a distinct difference between white and brown (whole-wheat) bread. Whole-wheat bread, with just the bran removed, has only eight percent of the whole wheat extracted. It therefore contains more vitamins, minerals, and protein than "enriched" white bread. But it still is far inferior to bread labeled "stone-ground, whole-grain," which can be found in health-food stores or in the health-food sections of most supermarkets.

Dr. Denis Burkitt, British physician and Nobel Laureate, wants white bread banished from human diets. World-famous for his research into the causes and treatment of cancer, he suspects the lack of bulk in white bread, among its other deficiencies, may have a link to certain types of cancers. James S. Turner wrote in *The Chemical Feast*, ". . . French-born nutritionist Dr. Jean Mayer thinks that America's white bleached dough products would not even be called bread in his native land. Their food value is almost zero."

Turner added that while only a small group of the necessary and natural nutrients are returned to white bread, "Currently the FDA food standards permit *93* ingredients—few of them nutrients—to be added to bread products at the discretion of the processors." Some of these additives may be hazardous to health.

The American Diet and the Need for Education in Nutrition

5

Australopithecus, an apelike creature regarded as one of man's early ancestors, probably ate a more nutritious diet fifteen million years ago than the average American eats today.

Australopithecus was one of the first animals to use weapons for hunting. (Before this creature, man's forerunners were vegetarians.) He supplemented his meat diet with roots, nuts, berries, and fruits, from which he received his necessary carbohydrates. Australopithecus ate what he needed, a diet high in protein, moderate in fat, and low in carbohydrates.

The average American today knows where to find sugar: *everywhere*. It is in his soft drinks, canned juices, baked goods, and even hidden in his breakfasts, lunches, and dinners. And just under twenty pounds of candy (almost pure sugar) per capita were consumed in America last year.

Americans have managed to turn primitive man's adequate nutrition 180 degrees around until it has become inadequate in protein, and high in fats and carbohydrates.

Drs. Louis N. Katz, Jeremiah Stamler, and Ruth Pick of Michael Reese Hospital, Chicago, wrote of the reversal:

"[Recent American diets] are . . . markedly different in composition . . . from any ever consumed by wild animals or most pre-literate peoples. [Today's] nutritional patterns . . . go back only about 8,000 years. Prior to that time, man had been exclusively a food gatherer. He had not yet learned to be a food producer. Inevitably, therefore, his eating habits differed markedly from ours. Composed of a variety of natural unprocessed foods, yielding a high ratio of essential nutrients to calories, his diets were invariably well nourishing and well balanced. . . .

"In the Fertile Crescent of the Middle East, man made the decisive historic leap from food gathering to food producing and became a farmer and herder. This Neolithic transition . . . made available for the first time many of the foods commonly consumed by most Americans today, . . . dairy products, eggs, cereals, breads. . . . In conjunction with industrialization, urbanization and the rise in per capita national income, 'richer' diets have become commonplace—diets containing sizable quantities of the more expensive high-fat foods of animal origin plus 'elegant' white bread and refined sugar. These foods are now consumed en masse in countries like the United States."

Australopithecus's body needed very little starch or sugar. This early man's genes passed from generation to generation, some changing only minutely through the ages, so modern man *still* needs relatively little sugar or starch. He can manufacture all that he requires from a nutritious diet. Thus, a problem: Man's ancient genetic design must absorb the average American's annual consumption of 250 pounds of refined sugar, flour, and cereals. It is no wonder that our metabolisms so often become imbalanced.

Our dietary "advances" may make commercialized foods look and taste better, but it is apparent that they cannot sustain good health. Health deficiencies have been created by the technology that gave the world's population so many advantages.

How bad is the American diet? America is not faced with

classical malnutrition—such as scurvy or severe beriberi—but does face a subclinical or subtle type that can have just as drastic an effect over a period of years.

Dr. Robert S. Goodhart of the National Vitamin Foundation wrote, ". . . Substantial proportions . . . of our population consume diets which fall short of the Recommended Dietary Allowances for viamin A, thiamine, riboflavin and ascorbic acid. . . . Many Americans of *all ages and socio-economic brackets* are subsisting on diets which fall substantially short of the RDA in respect to one or more essential nutrients." [Emphasis added]

The American food heritage consisted of the natural nutrients in meat, milk, cheese, fish, fruit, grains, nuts and vegetables. Even a decade or two ago, less attention was paid to processed foods and canned fish, fruits, and vegetables. Americans today eat *half* of their food processed in some way—canned, frozen, dehydrated, or milled. These foods are usually nutrient-deficient because of the processing.

A ten-state study of families in all income brackets by the Department of Health, Education and Welfare (HEW) completed in 1970 revealed that fifteen percent of all children surveyed showed evidence of growth retardation. Thirty-five to fifty-five percent of everyone studied suffered from one or more nutrient deficiencies. One-third of all children studied had anemia "to a degree that a pediatrician would prescribe therapy right away." One-third of all children studied had vitamin A deficiency.

HEW's evaluation: "The nutrition of a significant proportion of the American public is inadequate and has become worse."

Malnutrition is not confined to poor Americans. The affluent are just as likely to be deficient in minerals and vitamins, not because they cannot afford essential foods, but because they do not know what to eat or in what proportion.

Dr. George Christakis, head of the nutrition program of New York's Mount Sinai medical school, reports, ". . . About two-thirds of the nation's public-health and chronic-disease problems are related to how our fellow citizens eat. . . ." Dr. Tom Spies, formerly of Northwestern medical school, Chicago, suggested that the average American is eating just enough of the B-complex vitamins to prevent the development of severe symptoms of both beriberi and pellagra. HEW's nutritional survey learned that five percent of the population it studied had goiter, an iodine deficiency. It also found rickets, a vitamin D deficiency thought to have been eliminated in this country a generation ago.

In a 1973 series on nutrition, the *New York Times* called nutritionists who argue for vitamin supplementation "insurance-minded," implying these nutritionists wanted something extra in our nutrient intake, something not needed. Malnutrition in the United States is already so severe that these men are seeking something not extra at all. They are fighting an epidemic, an epidemic found in a host of deficiency-caused diseases now widespread among Americans.

The average American eats only a small percentage of the nutrient-containing foods necessary to sustain health and a normal sugar-regulating mechanism. A western university recently compiled "the most popular adult diet in the United States." Examine the sample menu shown below that was derived from this diet; it illustrates the gross imbalance, in most American diets, in favor of useless starches and away from nutrients and proteins. Then compare this diet with the sample 2000-calorie Nutrition-Wise Daily Menu (see Appendix II for other menus). The tables that follow these menus show the nutrient totals of the most popular U.S. diet and those of the 2000-calorie Nutrition-Wise daily menu and how each compares percentage-wise with the U.S. Government recommended dietary allowance (RDA).

MOST POPULAR ADULT DIET IN THE UNITED STATES

	CARB.	PROT.	FAT	TOTAL
		Cal.		
Breakfast				
Coffee and donuts				
(cream and sugar)	160	20	150	330
Snacks				
Coffee and sweet roll				
(cream and sugar)	140	25	70	235

	CARB.	PROT.	FAT	TOTAL
		Cal.		
Lunch				
2 hot dogs	10	60	180	250
Pickles	10	5	5	20
Soft drink	80	0	0	80
Apple Pie (small slice)	210	10	115	335
Snack				
Coffee and sweet roll				
(cream and sugar)	140	25	50	215
Dinner				
Meatballs (3 small)	45	50	175	270
Spaghetti (1 cup)	175	30	10	215
Green beans (½ cup)	10	5	0	15
Chopped salad	25	10	5	40
Chocolate cake	75	5	30	110
French Bread	60	5	5	70
Late Snack				
Coffee (cream and sugar)	20	0	25	45
Cookies (2)	150	10	60	220
TOTAL	1,310	260	880	2,450
	(51%)	(11%)	(38%)	

2000-CALORIE NUTRITION-WISE MENU

	CARB.	PROT.	FAT	TOTAL
		Cal.		
Breakfast				
3 apricot halves, stewed				
(noncalorically sweetened)	55	5	—	60
½ cup rice, cooked (whole grain)	85	10	—	95
1 egg plus 1 egg white, scrambled				
with	—	40	50	90
1 tbsp. nonfat dry milk solids	15	10	—	25

	CARB.	PROT.	FAT	TOTAL
		Cal.		
1 tbsp. wheat germ	10	5	—	15
2 tbsp. water	—	—	—	—
¼ tsp. brewer's yeast	—	—	—	—
3 oz. dried or chipped beef	—	115	50	165
1 slice whole-wheat bread	45	10	5	60
1 tsp. butter or margarine	—	—	35	35
1 glass (8 oz.) skim milk	50	35	—	85
TOTALS	260	230	140	630

Lunch

	CARB.	PROT.	FAT	TOTAL
1 cup consomme	—	35	—	35
1 envelope unflavored gelatin	—	30	—	30
6 oz. white fish, broiled	—	160	20	180
½ cup mustard greens	10	5	—	15
1 hard-cooked egg white	—	15	—	15
½ cup lima beans with pimento	65	20	—	85
1 slice whole-wheat bread	45	10	5	60
Lemon pudding	40	20	40	100
1 glass (8 oz.) skim milk	50	35	—	85
TOTALS	210	330	65	605

Dinner

	CARB.	PROT.	FAT	TOTAL
Salad: 1 med. tomato, stuffed with ½ cup cottage cheese and	25	5	5	35
1 tsp. chopped parsley	10	90	5	105
New England Boiled Dinner	75	165	105	345
Celery sticks (¼ stalk)	5	—	—	5
1 slice whole-wheat bread	45	10	5	60
Dessert: Molded fruit salad, made with				
1 envelope gelatin (unflavored)	—	30	—	30
¾ cup water	—	—	—	—

		CARB.	PROT.	FAT	TOTAL
			Cal.		
2 tbsp. lemon juice		10	—	—	10
½ cup fruit cocktail, nonca- lorically sweetened		45	—	—	45
1 glass (8 oz.) skim milk		50	35	—	85
	TOTALS	265	335	120	720
Before Bedtime					
½ glass (4 oz.) skim milk		25	20	—	45
	TOTALS	760	915	325	2,000
		(38%)	(45%)	(16%)	

RECOMMENDED DIETARY ALLOWANCE
BASED ON ADULT MALE 154 POUNDS

2800 Total Daily Calories

CA.	PHOS.	IRON	SOD.	POT.	A	B₁	B₂	NIA.	C	D
		mg.			*IU*			*mg.*		*IU*
800	800	10	—	—	5000	1.4	1.7	18	60	—

MOST POPULAR ADULT DIET IN THE UNITED STATES

2450 Total Daily Calories

CA.	PHOS.	IRON	SOD.	POT.	A	B₁	B₂	NIA.	C	D
		mg.			*IU*		*mg.*			*IU*
487	1158	13.6	3605	1452	2400	0.90	1.44	16.94	T	T

PERCENTAGE OF RECOMMENDED DIETARY ALLOWANCE
IN MOST POPULAR ADULT DIET

CA.	PHOS.	IRON	SOD.	POT.	A	B₁	B₂	NIA.	C	D
60%	145%	136%	—	—	40%	60%	80%	90%	—	—

NUTRITION-WISE MENU

2000 Total Daily Calories

CA.	PHOS.	IRON	SOD.	POT.	A	B₁	B₂	NIA.	C	D
		mg.			*IU*		*mg.*			*IU*
2165	3475	30.3	8600	6015	14,195	462	23.40	102.31	195	85

PERCENTAGE OF RECOMMENDED DIETARY ALLOWANCE
IN NUTRITION-WISE MENU

CA.	PHOS.	IRON	SOD.	POT.	A	B₁	B₂	NIA.	C	D
270%	435%	300%	—	—	280%	330%	135%	565%	320%	—

NOTE: T indicates a trace amount of the vitamin only;
      — indicates no available information from RDA

You can see that the Nutrition-Wise program is high in protein and essential nutrients and low in carbohydrates and fat. And while the recommended dietary allowance totals might sustain an American on a day-to-day basis, they are hardly enough to restore a state of metabolic equilibrium and a feeling of peak energy after years of bad eating and functional breakdown.

Beware of chemical additives. Food additives have become prevalent in American diets because they preserve, color, texturize, and flavor the increasing number of processed and refined foods in our stores. Such compounds as the preservative BHA (butylated hydroxyanisole) are given the GRAS (generally recognized as safe) label by the FDA, but no one really knows how safe or unsafe they may be. More than 485 million dollar's worth of additives went into American food in 1970, 150 million into artificial flavoring alone. It has been estimated that each American ate about five pounds of additives that year. Some of these chemicals may be partly responsible for the abnormal levels of insulin found in diabetic and hypoglycemic patients. Additives have no nutritional value, and they may actually be harmful.

Dr. Ben F. Feingold of the Kaiser Permanante Medical Center, San Francisco, told a 1973 American Medical Association convention that food additives may trigger extreme hyperactivity and severe learning disorders in children. Dr. Feingold took a group of San Francisco students who were suffering hyperactivity, short attention spans, and an inability to learn and placed them on a diet of additive-free, natural foods. He eliminated all artificial flavors and coloring, chemicals previously found in large quantities in their diets. Some of the children improved dramatically within several weeks.

Michael F. Jacobson, author of *Eater's Digest, The Consumer's Factbook of Food Additives,* reported that additives such as tannic acid (found in butter, caramels, and fruit) and sodium nitrite and nitrate (preservatives in many foods) may cause cancer. Others are linked to birth defects in animal studies, yet all are still on store shelves in large quantities.

The threat of infection has given way to the threat of cell starvation. The average American has been so carefully informed about bacterial and viral diseases that these no longer pose a threat. "Today germs are not our principal enemy," said Dr. Tom Spies. "Our chief medical adversary is . . . a disturbance of the inner balance of the constituents of our tissues, which are built from and maintained by necessary chemicals in the air we breathe, the water we drink and the food we eat.

"For a generation we have worked on the concept that our cells are never static and that in time they must be replaced in varying degrees by the nutrients obtained from food. More specifically, our working hypothesis has been that all disease is chemical and when we know enough about it, then it [will be] chemically correctable."

"If all that we know about nutrition were applied to modern society," Dr. Frank G. Boudreau wrote in the Department of Agriculture's *Food, the Yearbook of Agriculture,* "the result would be an enormous improvement in public health, at least equal to that which resulted when the germ theory of infectious disease was made the basis of public health and medical work."

The food industry must be held accountable. A Louis Harris poll completed in 1973 found that more than half of all adults questioned received their nutritional information—or misinformation—from advertising in magazines, newspapers, radio, or television.

"[The problem also] is not [just] the quality of food, . . . but the kinds of foods we eat," says Dr. Myron Winick, director of Columbia University's Institute of Human Nutrition. "Our choices are not nutritional choices, but instead are governed by a constant barrage of advertising and the speed of supermarket turnover.

"The food industry doesn't compete on the basis of the nutritive quality of the product it's selling, and the profit motive in selling and packaging is not always compatible with the best nutrition."

Cost plays a major part in what goes into America's food. Thirty years ago, the United States rid itself of rickets by not charging the consumer for vitamin D fortification in milk, but milk fortified with vitamin D is often sold today at premium prices, so many poor people simply do not buy it—and rickets has returned. Mentioned earlier was the U.S. Department of Health, Education and Welfare finding that five percent of the population it studied had goiter. Iodine uniformly added to salt will alleviate the symptoms of goiter and reduce the incidence of this disorder. It can be added to salt at a cost of one-fourth of a cent per year per person, but it is not added to all salt. Forty percent of the food markets in one statewide survey failed to stock *any* salt that was iodized. Kelp, which contains iodine plus many other materials, is even better.

These food-industry practices may save companies millions of dollars, but they are slowly eroding the national health. Soybean meal is a good source of protein and can be made to taste very much like meat. Indeed, it is now being sold at some meat counters. But it still lacks many of the nutrients found in meat. Also, the processing used to make soybeans look and taste like meat may change essential molecular structure, and therefore may affect the body's ability to utilize the available nutrients. The Food and Drug Administration should examine this possibility. If the past record of the food industry is any indication, the industry will not correct this situation if it exists, nor will it balance the soy product with a corresponding amount of the missing meat nutrients. The average American will fall further into a dietary deficiency gap. With each downward step, his health will grow worse.

A federal task force studied malnutrition in 1972 and suggested that improving the American diet might: reduce heart disease by one-quarter, reduce respiratory illness and infection by a fifth, reduce the death rate for pregnant women and newborn infants by half, reduce congenital birth defects by half, cut the number of severe geriatric difficulties by ten million, reduce arthritis by eight million, and add six years to the average black American's life.

Good nutrition is a matter of education. Only about half of America's housewives can come reasonably close to describing a nutritionally balanced meal. Yet eighty to ninety percent of these women *think* they supply their families with adequate nutrition. America's malnutrition stems not from lack of food, but from lack of nutritional knowledge. "Hunger can be solved with money, but only education can solve the problem of malnutrition," notes Dr. Dorothy Whipple, professor of pediatrics at Georgetown University.

In the analysis of the American diet presented earlier in this chapter, we can see that the average American does not know his nutritional friends from his nutritional enemies. And how is he to learn?

One of the most remarkable learning methods is simply to compare foods. For example, if we knew the poor nutrient value of most dry cereals—doubly bad because, in addition to the scarcity of nutrients, virtually all contain relatively large amounts of sugar—as compared with other foods, we would soon stop eating those useless products. Cats get a better meal out of their commercial cat food than do children who eat a product such as a well-known rice-based cereal.

A ⅝-ounce box of this breakfast cereal contains one gram of protein, fifteen grams of carbohydrates, and no fat. Its ingredients are: milled rice, sugar (the second largest ingredient in the package), salt and malt flavoring with sodium ascorbate, vitamins C, A, B_1, B_2, niacin, D, B_6, folic acid, iron phosphate, and preservatives.

An impressive list. But the vitamins supply only these percentages of the U.S. recommended dietary allowance: protein, two percent; vitamin A, fifteen percent; vitamin C, fifteen percent; niacin, fifteen percent; calcium, zero; iron, six percent; vitamin D, six percent; vitamin B_6, fifteen percent; folic acid, fifteen percent.

Purina Dairy Dinner for cats contains thirty-four ingredients, most of them nutrients. These are just a few of the ingredients those pets get: poultry by-product meal, soybean meal, dried whey, isolated soy protein, dried skim milk, dried brewers' yeast, dried whole egg, iodized salt, wheat-germ meal, phosphoric acid, choline chloride, B_{12} supplement, riboflavin, vitamin A, menadione sodium bisulfate (a source of vitamin K), vitamin E, thiamine, calcium pantothenate, niacin, ferrous sulfate, manganese sulfate, manganous oxide, zinc and copper oxides, and cobalt carbonate. *The meal is thirty percent protein.*

I am not recommending that children eat cat food. I am only noting the fact that our pets may be eating better than our children, so many of whom start their morning with a box of cold cereal, milk, and a glass of orange juice.

Thus, the need for more educational programs in nutrition. But obstacles exist: chiefly apathy. The food industry has done little to increase the nutritional value of many of its products primarily because the public has not demanded higher quality. Government agencies have not assumed the responsibility they should have borne in enforcing the production of better foods.

Proper nutrition simply means to eat "good" foods—those that supply our cells with the vital nutrients they need in regulated amounts—and to avoid harmful foods—those, like sugar, which can be linked to some disease state and those laced with chemical additives which used to be called adulterants.

For the hypoglycemic, nutrition is all-important. It is one of the few factors that he can control to improve his condition. The hypoglycemic's diet, therefore, must be extraordinarily strict. But what's good for the hypoglycemic is often compatible with general good nutrition.

Sugar *must not* be eaten by the hypoglycemic; but nonhypoglycemics should not eat sugar either. Foods rich in proteins, vitamins, minerals, amino acids, and unsaturated fatty acids should be substituted. Once these are substituted, sweets and starches tend to become less appetizing. Because sugar and starches are composed mostly of high-caloric carbohydrates, Nutrition-Wise programs make it possible to eat more nutrients while absorbing fewer calories.

Studies with animals have demonstrated the benefits of good nutrition. Controlled weight gain, the ability to reproduce, longevity (although studies have shown that rats that eat too much food have shorter lives), vitality, and stamina are all increased when animals eat a highly nutritious diet. The hypoglycemic human loses these same traits when he is poorly nourished.

I have noted previously that the chronic, degenerative diseases are rising in number critically, that good nutrition can ameliorate these diseases to some extent, and that Americans eat poorly. Yet *Consumer Reports* in 1970 wrote that "healthy people who eat balanced diets don't need [vitamin supplements]." The statement in itself is only partly correct. But the article fails to make clear that literally *millions* of Americans are not "healthy people who eat balanced diets." It does not mention that some people have poor genetic patterns and thus have greater nutritional needs. The truly disheartening fact is that most Americans do not even know of their deficiencies and they do not realize that such an inane statement as that made in *Consumer Reports* serves to absolve the food industry of its shortcomings.

Poor nutrition can make a middle-aged man old: his hair will turn gray, his teeth will rot, his skin will wrinkle and turn sallow, his eyes will glaze and cloud, his senses will become less acute, and, tragically, his memory will fade as more and more brain cells die.

Brain cells cannot be reproduced. They begin to die in all of us once adulthood is reached. But the rate at which they die is influenced heavily by the nutrients they receive. A forty-year-old man or woman who eats well and loses a thousand brain cells a day, a relatively paltry amount, will keep his or her mental acuity far longer than his or her malnourished counterpart who loses ten thousand or more cells daily.

Proper nutrition may have an effect on cancer. Although cultures in which cancers are relatively rare often have varying diets, these diets do contain similarities: They are well balanced and lacking in nonnutritious foods (notably sugar). Cooking time for most foods is kept to a minimum, and there is minimal use of large amounts of condiments, such as salt. And these cultures add virtually no preservatives or dyes to their foods. Most of the additives used in the American food industry have never been tested for their carcinogenic—or any other possible long-range harmful—effect.

A wide variety of such chemicals have been proved to be, or may yet be proved to be, carcinogens. An extract of sassafras, safrole, was used in root beer until 1960, when it was discovered to cause liver cancer. Oil of calamus was taken off the market as a natural flavoring in 1967 when it was found to cause intestinal tumors. DES (diethylstilbestrol), a food additive and synthetic female hormone that has been added to as much as seventy-five percent of the beef cattle in the United States to fatten them, has been known since 1938 to cause cancers in rats, but the additive was banned only last year. In the meantime, daughters of women treated with DES twenty years ago are now developing an uncommon cancer. The disease was caused by DES while the children were still in their mothers' wombs.

Other possible carcinogens that require more testing but are still on the market are the sweetener saccharin; the additive tannin, found in coffee, tea, and cocoa; the food coloring violet 1, used for meat inspection stamps and for candy and beverage coloring; the food coloring citrus 2, found in the skins of some oranges and tangerines; the food coloring red 2, used in cosmetics and a great many food products. In all these cases, animal studies have shown at least some carcinogenic results.

Sodium nitrite in meats and cold cuts prevents the growth of botulism bacteria, but it is now also considered a carcinogen by many researchers. When a nitrite compound combines with substances found in all meats and many other foods, called amines, it forms nitrosamine. "The nitrosamines [are] the best group of carcinogens," notes Dr. Samuel Epstein, professor of pharmacology at Case Western Reserve medical school. "The vast majority produce cancer." The Center for Science in the Public Interest, a professional group, charged that "both the Food and Drug Administration and the U.S. Department of Agriculture are dragging their feet on decisions to ban [nitrite food additives]."

Dr. Jacobson, the *Eater's Digest* author and a biologist at the Center, says that bacon is "the most dangerous food in the supermarket," because of the large amounts of nitrite and nitrate found in it. A cancer researcher at Oak Ridge National Laboratory, Dr. William Lijinsky, no longer eats meat or fish with nitrite in it. "I don't allow it in my house either," says Dr. Lijinsky.

The foods Americans eat also have an effect on birth defects. "According to the National Foundation-March of Dimes, every year 250,000 American babies are born with such defects as a cleft palate, club foot, or an open spine," writes Dr. Jacobson. "The National Foundation estimates that environmental factors, such as food additives, drugs, smoking, and pollution contribute to eighty percent of the birth defects." He also suggests that caffeine and quinine may be capable of producing such defects, but no one knows. Adequate tests have never been undertaken.

Food producers and suppliers are now required to write the amounts of calories, vitamins, minerals, and protein contained in their processed foods on labels. This type of labelling allows the consumer to plan meals that supply adequate numbers of nutrients in proper proportions. But it is far from complete. Although sugar, when used in a product, must be listed as an ingredient, the amount is rarely noted.

Labeled food is only part of the solution. People have to be made aware that diets must be regulated carefully by experts. If it is true, as Dr. C. S. Chlouverakis, director of the Obesity and Lipid Abnormalities Service at Buffalo's E. J. Meyer Memorial Hospital, suggests, that "it is likely that the dieting population [those who have tried to lose weight at least once by food regulation] represents the majority of the adult population in America, . . ." then there are a vast number of adults who are deprived of the nutrients they need and must be taught to distinguish between an adequate and inadequate weight-loss diet. No one diet is good for everyone; different people require different solutions. Each individual has a different metabolism and therefore different nutritional requirements. Two thousand years ago Lucretius, Roman poet and philosopher, noted: "What is food to one man may be fierce poison to others."

Regulate your nutritional intake. The application of the nutritional guidelines in the appendixes of this book will play a large part in the regulation of blood-sugar levels. But the menus and recipes included are meant to be adapted to the specific needs of individuals. An adequate daily caloric intake is determined by age, weight, sex, and a certain degree of trial and error. Generally speaking, among adults who are neither underweight nor overweight, males require about 20 calories per day for each pound of body weight and females 15 calories per pound of body weight. Older people must reduce their total caloric intake, and, because their recuperative powers diminish with age, their ratio of protein over carbohydrates and fats must be increased. Teen-agers also need more protein than the average adult.

The variety of menu plans listed in Appendix II will enable you to tailor meals to your own particular metabolic and caloric needs. Determine the daily calorie total appropriate for you and vary it until you find the range that keeps you feeling fit and satisfied. Keep in mind that calories are only one part of the total picture. Cheese, for example, has always been considered a good source of protein, and it is, yet the ratio of fat calories to protein in cheese is nearly three to one.

Also included in the nutritional charts of Appendix I are commonly eaten foods and in Appendix II the percentages the meals contain of the U.S. recommended dietary allowances for proteins, fats, and carbohydrates. However, bear in mind that the caloric, vitamin, and mineral values listed are only approximate; food is affected by soil conditions, transportation, storage, processing, and cooking.

Recommendations that may be useful to the hypoglycemic patient (or the nonhypoglycemic who truly wants to do something to keep himself healthy) follow:

1. Plan menus for a week's worth of meals at a time to make shopping more selective and less time-consuming.

2. *Never* buy foods that should be avoided; they can't be tempting if they're not around the house. If bought for others, store the forbidden provisions out of sight.

3. Buy as many natural, unprocessed foods as possible. Read labels and become familiar with the dietetic food section of your grocery store.

4. Plan variety-filled meals. Don't eat only leaf vegetables and meats, but diversify your nutritional program to include dairy products, fish, fowl, eggs, fruits, root vegetables, and such fungi as yeast or mushrooms. Diversification also means that you should eat more than animal muscle when you eat meat. Brain, liver, skin, and fat tissues all help round out your nutritional intake.

5. Weigh food portions to evaluate the calories and nutrients they contain. With a little practice you'll be able to estimate weights with an acceptable degree of accuracy.

6. Record daily food intake. This will help you overcome the temptations of empty, malignant calories and better evaluate the nutrients you're getting.

7. Don't attempt to cut down on total calories until metabolic balance has been restored and symptoms of hypoglycemia have abated.

8. Eat between-meal snacks to help regulate and stabilize blood-sugar levels. Consult the snack suggestions in the Appendix.

9. Use honey for sinking spells during the day or night, but use it sparingly. Add a small amount to a glass of orange juice or milk if you feel especially sluggish before breakfast.

10. Compensate for eating processed carbohydrates (flour and sugar products) with increased dosages of vitamins and minerals. Predigested protein in liquid form is a good source of amino acids. This form of protein is available at drugstores, health-food stores, and special departments in discount or department stores.

11. Adopt a positive attitude toward your Nutrition-Wise program. Don't feel sorry about that missed piece of pie or glass of soda pop. Rather, concentrate on the detrimental effects of such foods.

12. Don't be afraid to stand by your nutritional convictions when dining in a restaurant. If it is a reputable establishment, it will gladly accommodate special requests.

13. *Avoid:* sugar-sweetened beverages and fruit juices, canned fruits in syrup, frozen fruits with sugar, molasses, sugar-laden snacks, convenience foods and desserts, alcoholic beverages, tea, coffee (except decaffeinated), whole milk, chocolate milk, bacon, pork, dried beans, cereals, cheese (except low-fat varieties), cream, butter, crackers, white bread, rice, rolls, biscuits, pizza, noodles, macaroni products, potatoes, pastries, pies, cakes, candies, ice cream, sherbet, creamed foods, gravies.

Becoming nutrition-wise involves learning not only what to avoid but what to add to your diet and how to do it conveniently and effectively. One trick is to supplement your eating with nutrition boosters. These are included here, together with the everyday foods to which they may be added.

Brewers' yeast. Overcome the deficiencies of both processed and unprocessed foods by adding nutrient-rich brewers' yeast to as many foods as possible. Add brewers' yeast to: vegetable juices, soups, hamburgers, meat loaf, cereals, sandwich spreads, milk drinks, gravies, baked beans, applesauce, Spanish rice, meat, stews and hashes, cakes, cookies, muffins, pancakes, waffles, breads, biscuits (including all mixes).

Brewers' yeast may be purchased in powder or tablet form at groceries, drugstores, and health-food stores. Use as directed.

Powdered milk. Powdered skim milk contains over thirty-six percent protein of high biologic value. You can increase your protein, natural vitamins, and minerals and avoid the animal fat of whole milk by adding skim milk solids to your food as follows:

Scrambled eggs: *1 tablespoonful per egg.*
Custards, sauces, puddings: *Add 1 tablespoonful to the liquid in the recipe.*
Hamburger, meat loaf, and meat balls: *2 tablespoonfuls to each portion.*
Clear, canned, and homemade soups: *1 or 2 tablespoonfuls per bowl.*
Cooked cereals: *1 or 2 tablespoonfuls per serving.*
Gravies (no fat): *1 or 2 tablespoonfuls for thickening.*
Bread, cakes, muffins, cookies, pancake recipes, and mixes: *1 or 2 tablespoonfuls to standard recipe.*

Cottage cheese. This will be one of your best friends when you become nutrition-wise. A cup of cottage cheese yields slightly over 200 calories, most of them protein. You would have to drink 2½ pints of whole milk to get the same amount of protein, but you would also get over four times as many total calories. And, about half of these would be fat calories.

A cup of cottage cheese (noncreamed) contains only 10 fat calories. An equal amount (in weight) of pork sausage (patties or links) contains 900 fat calories, or ninety times as much.

Cottage cheese can be used in these ways:

Add it to ground or chopped nuts, olives, onions, chives, pimento, chopped celery, chopped green or red peppers, shredded carrots, diced apples, dietetic jelly or preserves, chopped pickles, chopped or sliced hard-boiled eggs, chopped ham, leftover liver, liver paste, or diced dried beef for sandwich combinations.

Add cottage cheese to sauces, puddings, mayonnaise, salad dressings.

Use cottage cheese as a topping on gelatin and other molded desserts.

Add 1 tablespoon of cottage cheese for each egg to be scrambled. Add chipped beef, diced ham, or ground beef, and scramble the eggs.

Combine cottage cheese with spiced peaches or apple rings for a good accompaniment to meat or poultry dishes.

Whip cottage cheese in a tomato or bouillon aspic.

Heap cottage cheese onto honeydew, casaba, or cantaloupe halves for breakfast, or as a first or last course for main meals.

Use cottage cheese as the base for a cooked sauce over Brussels sprouts, asparagus, broccoli, boiled onions, green beans, and carrots.

Fill big ripe, red tomatoes or green pepper halves with cottage cheese for added protein calories. Serve cottage cheese as a main dish, seasoned with vinegar, cinnamon, nutmeg, or favorite herbs and spices. Top with slivered almonds or lemon juice.

Add cottage cheese to any sauces and salad dressings to proteinize them.

Blend cottage cheese with lemon juice, buttermilk, or yogurt for a low-calorie, high protein, nutrition-wise sour cream.

Combine low-calorie jams, jellies, or preserves with cottage cheese for your breakfast toast.

Enhance the flavor and nutrient value of a dish of cottage cheese with honey and wheat germ for a light lunch.

Pile cottage cheese on pieces of pineapple, sliced halved peaches, or apricots for added protein calories.

Try a cottage cheese omelet, or fill pancakes with cottage cheese and low-calorie jam or preserves for a festive and nutritious brunch.

Add cottage cheese to pancakes, muffins, cakes, and cookies to step up your protein calories.

Whip cottage cheese with butter flavoring and saffron for coloring for a low-calorie spread. Vegetable oil may be added.

Whip cottage cheese into butter or margarine to increase its protein content.

Use cottage cheese, whipped and seasoned, as a baked potato topper.

Use cottage cheese, gelatin, and noncaloric sweetener to make a low-calorie cheesecake (see recipe in Appendix III).

Use cottage cheese as a base for raw vegetable dips.

Top fish, seafood, beef, veal, chicken, or turkey with whipped and seasoned cottage cheese.

Use cottage cheese as you would cream cheese in cake or muffins, toppings or frostings, cocktail spreads, and molded salads.

Whip cottage cheese with canned evaporated skim milk and sweeten with noncaloric artificial sweetener to taste for use as a substitute for whipped cream.

Fresh or canned orange juice and other fruit juices can flavor cottage cheese dishes.

Mix 1 cup of cottage cheese with chopped nuts, celery, diced green peppers, raisins, pimento, chopped olives, or diced hard-boiled eggs for tasty variety.

Gelatin. Unflavored gelatin is another nutritional friend. It is all protein. However, it lacks the essential amino acid tryptophan, and should be mixed or eaten with some animal protein for full effectiveness.

Do not confuse unflavored gelatin with the sweetened and flavored brand-name gelatins. They are eighty-five percent sugar.

Unflavored gelatin is excellent as a thickening agent. It can be used for all types of aspics, jellied soups, and consommes, or added, without jelling, to bouillon, tea, or coffee for a nutritious hot beverage.

Gelatin can be mixed with cold drinks, such as fruit juices, milk, and vegetable juices, but must be stirred and drunk quickly before it jells.

Add gelatin to puddings, custards, whips, fluffs, snows, and creams for healthier dessert dishes.

Liver. Liver is such a nutritious food that you should include it in your menu at least once or twice a week. It is an excellent source of protein and all of the B-complex vitamins. It is also a good source of vitamin A. Do not overcook it or it will lose its precious nutrients.

Dice or chop any kind of liver (beef, calf, pork, lamb, or chicken) and mix it into meat patties, meat loaf, or meatballs.

Grind cooked liver into a liver paste to use as a sandwich or cracker spread.

Liquefy a small amount of raw liver in a blender and add it to vegetable, fruit, or milk drinks.

If you don't care for cooked liver, substitute powdered dessicated liver, obtainable from drugstore or health-food store. Add a small amount to drinks, hamburgers, and meat loaves.

Wheat germ. Wheat germ is a rich source of unsaturated fatty acids, the B-complex vitamins, vitamin E, minerals, and protein. If it is processed or toasted, it loses most of its precious vitamin E, and if not kept refrigerated, will soon become rancid and unusable.

Fortify many of your foods and menus by using wheat germ in the following ways:

Cereals, hot or cold: *Add 1 tablespoonful to each portion.*
Soup: *Add 1 or 2 tablespoonfuls to each serving. Wheat germ can be used to thicken clear soups.*
Salads: *Add to taste to mixed green or molded salads.*
Hamburgers, meat loaf: *Add 1 or 2 tablespoonfuls per serving.*
Cream gravy: *2 tablespoonfuls of wheat germ.*
Vegetable juices: *Add 1 teaspoonful per 4-ounce glass.*

Soybean products. Soybeans contain all the essential amino acids in good proportions and are one of the few nonanimal proteins that are considered to be complete. They also contain lecithin, which helps to reduce high cholesterol levels in the blood.

Defatted soybean flour is considered high in digestibility, nearly as high as meat, eggs, and milk. It contains goodly amounts of iron, calcium, and other nutrient minerals and is high in vitamins.

Soy flour can be added to many foods to increase their nutritional content.

Add soy flour to wheat or rye flour for making bread. Since soy flour does not contain gluten (an elastic protein substance that gives cohesiveness to dough), it can only replace ten to twelve percent of the wheat or rye flour in bread recipes.

Soybean milk can be used by those who are allergic to cow's milk or for cardiac patients on low-sodium diets.

Soy cheese, or tofu, can be used as a good source of protein.

Vegetarians should include soybean products in their diets as substitutes for meat proteins.

Lecithin. Lecithin is a relatively tasteless water-soluble granular powder made from defatted soybeans. It is a component of all living cells and plays a vital role in the biochemistry of the body.

Lecithin is an emulsifying agent that tends to break up large fat globules into smaller droplets that can be utilized better by the body. It appears to have a cholesterol-lowering effect on patients with high blood-cholesterol levels. Cholesterol increases in the blood when lecithin levels drop.

Dr. Lester Morrison and his associates in Los Angeles have used lecithin as adjunctive therapy in the prevention and treatment of arteriosclerosis and heart conditions and find that it has great value in reducing high cholesterol levels.

Physicians who prescribe lecithin recommend 4 to 6 tablespoonfuls a day when cholesterol levels are high, and then 1 or 2 tablespoonfuls a day to maintain low levels and prevent the ravages of clogged arteries.

Use granular lecithin in milk and vegetable or fruit juices. Or add it to sandwich spreads.

Evaporated skim milk. The addition of canned evaporated skim milk to foods and beverages is a fast and easy way of stepping up their nutrient content. It is an excellent source of all of the proteins, minerals, and B-vitamins that occur in regular evaporated and whole milk, but without the fat (butterfat) calories. It differs from powdered milk only in water content.

Evaporated skim milk stores easily, keeps well, and is a convenient emergency food. It's a good idea to keep a supply of it on hand at all times.

Augment the protein, vitamin, and mineral content of these foods by using evaporated skim milk instead of regular evaporated or whole milk: scrambled eggs, hamburgers, meat loaf, meatballs, cooked cereals, dips, whips, appetizer spreads, sandwich spreads, molded salads, aspics, sauces, salad dressings, breads, waffles, pancakes, cakes, cookies, toppings, frostings, beverages, gravies, custards, and puddings.

An unattributed aphorism says, "Rules are meant for those expected to obey; principles for those who are expected to think." The suggestions and nutrition boosters here and the menus and recipes in the appendixes are for those who want to improve their nutritional principles. For the hypoglycemic, they are mandatory. For the aware layman, they are preventive.

Fight Disease Before It Happens:
The Power of Preventive Medicine

6

Preventive medicine is an *attitude* that can save many lives. Most simply, it combines nutritional fortification against disease with good health care and early detection of illness symptoms.

The key to preventive medicine lies in the control of the nutri-genetic factor. Those doctors who practice preventively do not wait for middle-aged men to have their heart attacks but treat all the adult male patients with heart disease prevention in mind. They give their female patients who are likely to bear children sound nutritional consulting and nutritional supplements when necessary, long before they become pregnant. When these women do conceive, the developing fetuses will enjoy the advantages of good nutrition.

Children born of nutritionally educated parents will be provided with good nutrition and proper instruction. Once on their own, they will eat properly because they have *learned* to eat properly. They will not be likely to become victims of chronic, degenerative diseases.

Support for this type of treatment is growing. A joint task group on nutrition of the Department of Agriculture and state universities and land-grant colleges, notes:

"Major health problems are diet-related. Most of the health problems underlying the leading causes of death in the United States could be modified by improvements in diet. . . .

"Most nutritionists and clinicians feel that the real potential from improved diet is preventive in that it may defer or modify the development of a disease state so that a clinical condition does not develop."

The U.S. General Accounting Office reported to Congress on November 20, 1972:

"Unless preventive medicine receives more attention, the nation's health care system may not be able to meet future demands."

The present health-care system in the United States is not geared toward prevention. The vast bulk of our health services and facilities are designed to treat illnesses and injuries only after they occur. The emphasis on curative treatment is indicated in health-care expenditures, medical education, insurance incentives, and socioeconomic conditions that fail to encourage preventive care.

As a nation, we boast about the money spent on medical health care. It is not *health* care at all, but *sick* care. We devote all our resources to treating people after they are already ill, rather than showing healthy people how to keep from getting sick in the first place. The average American family spends about two thousand dollars a year in doctors' fees and drugs. These costs could be reduced sharply merely by including adequate nutrition in preventive medical health care.

The reason for the high medical expenses is that preventive medicine is not practiced adequately; malnutrition and chronic diseases are engendered by mineral depleted soils. Devitalized, synthetic, and substitute foods are promoted constantly. Toxins such as herbicides and pesticides are still being eaten and absorbed by the body, and professionals and laymen alike have not been taught the truth about nutrition.

Dr. Willard A. Krehl told a symposium at the Massachusetts

Institute of Technology that "greater realization is needed in medicine and in public health that good nutrition along with good hygiene are the best weapons available in the prevention of disease. . . . The most important measure that could be taken to prevent the development of many chronic diseases would be the provision of consistently good individual nutrition, supervised by physicians with a strong assistance from the housewife, from conception to the grave."

"This country is rapidly becoming one that has never produced so much food and so little nutrition," consumer advocate Ralph Nader said recently. It is tragic to see good nutrition within the grasp of nearly all Americans yet bypassed by so many.

Good health depends on the body's resistance to disease. In medicine, this is known as host resistance. When a body's defenses are weak, it is more likely to develop disease. That is, when host resistance is low, the body has been biochemically imbalanced; this state precedes many of the diseases we try to cure today.

Despite these facts, doctors are still taught to heal the sick, not to prevent illness, but more and more physicians are voicing their disapproval. Said one: "The ideal of medicine is the prevention of disease, and the necessity for curative treatment is a tacit admission of failure."

Dr. George James, the late dean of Mount Sinai medical school, New York, noted: "Preventive medicine is not as fortunate as was the weather in Mark Twain's familiar statement. Not only are we doing very little about it, but we do not even talk about it very much. The lesson of history is that hardly any disease of major significance has ever been effectively controlled by attacking it only after symptoms have occurred. Why, therefore, this enormous enthusiasm for heroic surgery, coronary care units in hospitals and renal dialysis centers, concurrently with years of relative indifference to the curbing of cigarette smoking, lowering of dietary saturated fats, control of obesity and the detection and treatment of nonclinical hypertension, glaucoma, diabetes, and carcinoma [cancer] of the cervix?"

Curative medicine leads to an often-fatal waiting game. **Dr. Roger J.** Williams wryly describes the rules in *Nutrition Against Disease:*

"Wait until deformed and mentally retarded babies are born; then give them loving attention. Wait until heart attacks come; then, if the patient is still alive, give him or her the best care possible. Wait until mental disease strikes; then give considerate treatment. Wait until alcoholism strikes; then turn to the task of rehabilitation. Wait until cancer growth becomes apparent; then try to cut it out or burn it out with suitable radiation."

Colds can be prevented. The common cold is a near-perfect example of contrasting views among physicians in the growing battle between preventive and curative medicine.

The cold costs the American worker from $5 to $15 billion in lost wages each year. Most physicians recommend aspirin to ameliorate the cold's symptoms, although they know it does little to prevent the cold or even shorten its duration. And the drug, like any other, can be harmful. It can cause uncomfortable allergic reactions and it can contribute to the formation of duodenal ulcers. It is the single most common drug used in suicides, and it causes nearly fifteen percent of all poisoning deaths among children. Cold remedies often have other ingredients added to aspirin to give additional relief, and these drugs also can be dangerous. Americans spend $5,000,000 a year on cold remedies that do nothing for prevention.

But Dr. Linus Pauling, winner of the 1954 Nobel Prize in chemistry and winner of the 1958 Nobel Peace Prize, suggests that colds *can* be prevented without the use of drugs of any kind. Dr. Pauling's preventive technique—described in his book, *Vitamin C and the Common Cold,* published in 1970—is to use massive doses of ascorbic acid (vitamin C). If a cold has developed, Dr. Pauling says, vitamin C will lessen its strength and shorten its stay.

The vengeful response of many in the medical profession to Dr. Pauling's findings has left him an outcast. The man who has been called the "greatest of all chemists" by Nobel Laureate

J. D. Watson, one of the discoverers of the structure of DNA (the chemical building-block of life), and whose work constitutes a basic part of the foundation of molecular medicine, has suddenly found himself a medical renegade.

Dr. Charles C. Edwards, chief of the U.S. Food and Drug Administration, said, after Dr. Pauling's book on vitamin C was published: "There is no scientific evidence . . . that vitamin C is capable of preventing or curing colds." He refused to meet with Dr. Pauling to discuss the scientist's evidence.

On June 27, 1973, however, *Medical Tribune* reported: ". . . Studies from Europe and Canada have increasingly confirmed [Dr. Pauling's] views on vitamin C and the common cold [and] have indicated that vitamin C may be even more important than Dr. Pauling asserted."

And in January 1974, Dr. Geoffrey H. Bourne, an internationally known scientist whose specialty is vitamin deficiencies, announced that a growing accumulation of evidence confirms Dr. Pauling's theory that daily consumption of vitamin C prevents colds and lessens symptoms. Dr. Bourne edits the *World Review of Nutrition.*

Perhaps Dr. Pauling is now confronting the same obstacles faced by other visionaries in the past. Pasteur found the microbe. Freud discovered psychotherapy. Both were told their ideas were preposterous, but gradually their theories were endorsed, then adopted. Today, at the mercy of orthodox medicine's scorn, in addition to Dr. Pauling, are English psychiatrist R. D. Laing, with revolutionary theories on schizophrenia, and those men at Canada's Shute Clinic, who emphasize the tremendous importance of vitamin E in the maintenance of good health.

As long as nutrition—and vitamin C (ascorbic acid) is considered a nutritional supplement, not a drug—is not considered a major part of the curricula of medical schools, the medical attitude will continue to be one described and chastised in a lead editorial from *The American Journal of Public Health:* "We can, through a variety of expensive techniques, keep a few of the middle-aged and elderly alive for a few more precarious years, and yet we allow thousands of our young to die of diseases which we can easily and inexpensively prevent."

Why do so many physicians ignore hypoglycemia? Most physicians rarely consider a patient's nutrition. Because many physicians overlook this aspect, they rarely find malnourished or hypoglycemic patients. But the fact remains that most practicing physicians have such patients in their offices weekly.

And if doctors do discover a case of hypoglycemia, they do not recognize it as a serious and common problem, although the disease has been described repeatedly in medical journals since its discovery in 1924.

Why don't physicians consider hypoglycemia seriously? The problem begins in medical schools. Only 12 of the U.S. institutions have full departments of nutrition. Medical schools traditionally have been slow to innovate, slow to look for new answers to old problems, slow even to accept some *new* problems.

The medical school that does not educate its students in all aspects of good nutrition—and its relevance to good health, disease prevention, and longevity—is robbing the future doctor and his prospective patients of complete health care.

Doctors can do only what they have been trained to do. If their teaching is incomplete, their diagnostic technique when they enter practice will be incomplete as well. Medical school teachers each have their own priorities, and they do not want time devoted to nutrition at their expense. The eye, nose, and throat specialist wants more time for his specialty; the abdominal surgeon wants more time for his. The student "must" know more about neurology, more about cardiology.

Nutrition, a field that could help *all* these specialties, has little power within the medical school hierarchies, so it is largely ignored.

These same teaching physicians also have great influence outside their classrooms. Their research reports, published in medical journals, are often the determining factors in setting medical precedent for practicing physicians. These scientists regard the overall question of nutrition, and specifically low blood sugar, as a fad rather than a serious medical issue. They battle over diversionary issues, such as the amount of cholesterol in eggs, but cholesterol in eggs is not a problem. Nature put eggs together perfectly. They are a good food, probably the best food-dollar-buy today.

Practicing physicians are also enormously busy. The administration of a five- or six-hour glucose-tolerance test and the half-hourly blood sampling and analysis in the doctor's office, is time-consuming and tedious. How much simpler it is to prescribe a tranquilizer for an anxious patient and nitroglycerin pills for one suffering with anginal pains.

An additional barrier exists. Virtually all physicians are conservative in their work because they do not want to be considered different by their colleagues. They continue to prescribe a few relatively well-accepted medicines and continue to use orthodox methods to treat the acutely ill. They will not think outside the narrow channels that differentiate innovative treatment from orthodox. Most do not think of disease prevention, other than to give patients the necessary inoculations for various infectious diseases. They do not prevent mild deficiencies from becoming severe deficiencies, and few look for metabolic imbalances in otherwise healthy patients, even though the evidence is clear that such imbalances overlooked today will develop into the chronic, degenerative diseases that will have to be treated vigorously tomorrow.

A doctor in a large Texas hospital, one of the most respected physicians there, recently suffered a heart attack. He went to the famed Mayo Clinic for tests as well as to Canada's Shute Clinic. He returned convinced that vitamin E, today's most controversial nutrient supplement, could help him.

Most of the orthodox medical community consider vitamin E nearly worthless. Others, especially nutritionists, suggest vitamin E is of immeasurable help in cardiovascular ailments because it enables cells to accept oxygen more readily. It also seems to reduce the amount of fat circulating in the bloodstream and thus allows less fat buildup on arterial walls. It is this fat coating in many cases that causes heart attacks because the flow of blood to the heart is restricted.

The Texas physician now takes vitamin E regularly, but refuses to recommend it to his patients. His position at the hospital, he says, prevents him from doing so, but in reality, he simply does not want to be labeled a nonconformist.

Historically, cases of innovation-resistant physicians are legion.

In 1918, a young researcher working with patients suffering from pernicious anemia discovered that a liver extract he formulated had remarkably beneficial effects on his patients. Pernicious anemia is a condition in which the body fails to produce enough blood. Too few red blood cells means that too little oxygen, normally carried by these cells, reaches the body's tissues. The pernicious anemia victim is pallid, weak, often dizzy, fatigues easily, and, in more severe cases, is constantly bothered by an abnormal heartbeat and breathing pattern. When the researcher inoculated his patients with his new liver extract, the oxygen-carrying abiilty of their blood skyrocketed, and their fatigue lessened.

Within months, he could have isolated the nearly magical element in the extract and he would have discovered vitamin B_{12}. Instead, his labor was termed ridiculous. His positive results, he was told, were entirely coincidental cases of spontaneous remission; that is, his patients recovered "by themselves," without his aid.

The young researcher not only never completed his work, but left medical research altogether. An obviously creative scientist was lost, and pernicious anemia continued to strike victims who might have been helped.

A similar battle is waged by nutritionists concerned with hypoglycemia. "All too often one finds . . . nutritional status dismissed with the cursory statement that the patient is well-nourished and well-developed or that the patient seems to be getting a satisfactory diet," writes Dr. Willard A. Krehl formerly of the University of Iowa.

"It is reasonable to assume . . ." he says, "that nutritional deficiencies of all grades exist and do not necessarily appear as the . . . evidence of the classical deficiency diseases. . . . [A person] may have inadequate . . . nutritional status without overt evidence of nutritional disease; the deficits may begin early in life and continue for long periods of time. They may contribute ultimately to an illness without themselves becoming identified as the cause of or even related to the illness."

Dr. Krehl's words strike a key blow for the undiagnosed hypoglycemic. But even a doctor who does determine that a patient has hypoglycemia may still be reluctant to tell him. The disease has no cure. It cannot be treated with a drug that will send the patient home feeling well. Hypoglycemia can often be controlled with better eating and nutritional supplements, but the doctor must forbid the hypoglycemic to eat most of the carbohydrates—the candies, sodas, and desserts—he's lived on most of his life. It is easier to tell the patient that his fatigue is from overwork, that his migraine headaches should vanish with the muscle relaxers he will be given, or that his depression is related to his uneasy marriage.

When a patient is nervous, weak, and upset, he gets a tranquilizer rather than a test for hypoglycemia. The next month he returns, feeling a little better, but still not feeling quite "right." He may receive a shot of vitamin B_{12} or a prescription drug, but hypoglycemia is incredibly flexible. As soon as one aspect is treated, it is likely to create an entirely new symptom. The cycle continues, and the basic problem remains undetected and untreated.

Even while the doctor is examining a hypoglycemic, a medical journal in his morning mail may carry a report on the very symptoms his patient exhibits—correctly attributing them to hypoglycemia. Over five hundred published articles have been written since the disease was discovered, and medical journals have trebled in number since World War II. The physician, bombarded with massive quantities of literature, simply does not have time to read it all.

If a physician does have a chance to read—or better, attend a symposium—about hypoglycemia, he may still be misled.

Such a symposium was held in 1970 in Dallas. One of the speakers, a Philadelphia endocrinologist, related hypoglycemia's *sole* cause to tumors in the pancreas, the gland that produces the hormone insulin which, when secreted into the bloodstream, lowers the amount of blood sugar in the body. *These tumors are the rarest cause of hypoglycemia.* I have practiced for twenty-five years and have never seen one.

These "experts" mislead their colleagues by speaking of hypoglycemia as if it were some exotic, bizarre condition. It is one of the most common illnesses in the United States, and thousands of

Americans have forgotten, or perhaps have never known, what it is like to feel completely healthy.

Anything that stops the occurrence of disease is preventive medicine. Inoculations (close to half of all American children are not adequately immunized), annual checkups (two-thirds of the nation's children under fifteen receive inadequate health care), a clean environment, family planning, abstinence from smoking, and, most important, a sound nutritional plan all fall into this category.

I believe that a number of illnesses can be more effectively controlled, *and at far less cost,* by preventive medicine than by current attempts directed toward treatment and cure. These illnesses include some of the deadliest confronting Americans. They include all of the chronic, degenerative diseases, those that begin with a metabolic dysequilibrium that gradually upsets systemic balance. Preventive medicine checks any imbalance from building beyond controllable points, and keeps constant vigilance over the nutrigenetic factor.

Curative medicine sometimes arrives too late to help. Perhaps this is part of the reason that the United States is the only nation in the world that, according to the World Health Organization, has shown virtually no increase in life expectancy in recent years. The United States now ranks seventeenth among nations in life longevity.

If these statistics are to change, American physicians must learn to think more in terms of detection and less in terms of analysis of disease symptoms. Today, subclinical nutrient deficiencies are ignored.

What can preventive medicine do? If physicians and their patients tried supernutrition, good steady nutritional plans supplemented with vitamins and minerals often missing from American diets, there would be a decrease in the number of people suffering from ulcers, anemia, high blood pressure, kidney stones, coronary heart disease, stroke, gout, and obesity. It would also help slow natural aging processes.

Even diseases such as epilepsy, multiple sclerosis, muscular dystrophy, and cancer might be examined through preventive medicine's nutritional eye.

These possibilities do exist, but little money has been allocated publicly or privately to study nutritional effects. Research plays an important part in any preventive program, yet money has been hard to come by for many researchers because of a misdirection of priorities.

"There is literally nothing that will more surely improve the quality of American life than health research," wrote Dr. James T. Grace, Jr., former director of the Roswell Park Memorial Institute, Buffalo, New York. "Our only hope of really controlling devastating diseases and their enormous costs is through research. A cure of cancer, for example, would do more for our citizens than a thousand Regional Medical Programs—at a fraction of the cost—and it can come only through research."

The federal government finances virtually *all* scientific research. But since 1964, federal biomedical research spending has tapered off drastically, rising only about 2.5 percent a year while research costs have risen from 8 to 16 percent annually.

The long-range effects are graver than the termination of present research projects, closing of facilities, and scientists' loss of jobs would indicate. It takes ten to fifteen years to train a scientist, and experience shows that once a science student is forced to stop his studies, he does not usually return to them. Research teams and projects forced to disband do not magically reappear a year or two later when money is refunded for them. It is not that money is absent, either. Money to train these men and women is there, but the decision to divert it from other sources is not.

- Each American's share of defense spending in 1970 was $400. Each American's share of cancer research was $2.

- The United States spent $111 million in 1970 for research in mental illness, a problem that affects some twenty million Americans. In the same year it spent $187.5 million for outdoor recreation.

- One in six Americans now alive, a total of thirty-four million people, will die of cancer unless new cures are found. In 1973, 325,000 Americans died of cancer and one of four Americans now alive, fifty-one million people, will eventually have some form of the disease.

- We spend more each *day* on military matters than each *year* on medical research.

The public is entitled to the benefits of preventive medicine in all its varied aspects. But it is apparent that the public must demand knowledge from the food industries, the government, and the medical profession.

Medical science must use commonsense applications of all the available research it *does* have in combatting chronic, degenerative diseases. The physician must consider more than a symptom or a single diseased organ—he must think of the wholeness of man in relation to his environment.

But a comprehensive preventive campaign must do more than stimulate physicians. It must arouse the public from its lethargy to combat the irresponsibility of food and food-related industries.

If physicians and patients are to prevent the ravages of the greatest killers in the country, the chronic "breakdown" diseases, they must think in terms of positive health. Every person must develop a health conscience, become informed about his health and the health of those around him.

Schools and mass media are the primary conduits for instruction, but others are needed. Home health aides could teach nutrition and the benefits of prenatal care and nutrition classes could be held in neighborhood health centers.

But medical schools must play the basic role. They must change the attitudes of future doctors. (Many medical students are not waiting for curriculum change. Student groups in a number of medical schools are developing their own programs to take members into communities to see firsthand the need for preventive medicine. A growing number of medical schools—for example, Case Western Reserve, Mount Sinai, Albert Einstein, Yale—have begun to emphasize preventive medicine in their curricula.)

But medical schools have yet to proclaim their independence from the dollar influence of the food hierarchy. They *can* refuse grants, fellowships, and capital funds from these industries if the industries prevent the teaching of proper, optimum nutrition.

One completely independent, non-profit organization dedicated to research and education in the area of preventive medicine is the International Preventive Medicine Foundation, 871 Frostwood Drive, Houston, Texas 77024.

Perhaps the future will finally approximate Thomas Alva Edison's prediction: "The doctor of the future will give no medicine, but will interest his patients in the care of the human frame in diet and in the care and prevention of disease."

Hypoglycemia and Related Physical Disorders

7

Before the discovery of the hormone insulin in 1921, little hope could be offered to sufferers of diabetes; these unfortunate people had a life expectancy of only four or five years after the first appearance of the disease. Insulin—originally hailed as the diabetic's panacea—together with dietary control has helped to lengthen the diabetic's life, but he still lives only two-thirds as long as the average individual.

Insulin, like the other tools of symptomatic treatment, only ameliorates the effect of diabetes. It does not cure the disease. The control of the diabetic's sugar level with insulin does not prevent the associated problems that the disease carries with it. It is not the answer to the patient's metabolic imbalance, basic to the development of the disease.

Diabetics suffer from coronary heart disease at a rate twice that of nondiabetics. Hardening of the arteries occurs more often. The smaller blood vessels throughout the body deteriorate ceaselessly.

The gradual damage of these smaller vessels is likely to affect nearly every organ, tissue, or gland in the body.

For example, deterioration in the blood vessels of the eye as a result of diabetes can cause blindness. In 1947, only four percent of all blindness was attributed to this cause. Today, that figure is twenty-two percent. A New York ophthalmologist reports that diabetic retinopathy, the medical term for this arterial disease, rivals glaucoma as the leading cause of blindness.

Kidney failure and muscular, nervous, and skin disorders are also associated with diabetes, according to investigators.

Diabetes is more widespread than is commonly believed. The disease ranks sixth as a cause of death in the United States. The mortality rate may be far higher, however, because it does not include the cardiovascular or circulatory diseases from which the undiagnosed diabetic may die.

Some surveys suggest that about 2.3 million Americans have diabetes today. Other researchers argue 1.6 million more have the disease without knowing it. These figures are far too low. Once the nutrigenetic factor is accepted as the basis of metabolic dysequilibrium, many more cases will be uncovered.

"There is an even greater total of suspects who are *progressing into* diabetes," notes Dr. Glen McDonald of the U.S. Public Health Service. "In one large Public Health Service screening program, 10 percent of an unselected adult population were found positive." Chicago's Jackson Park Hospital, with others of the city's medical institutions, has been testing all patients for diabetes. Doctors there found diabetes in six percent of those tested; another twenty-seven percent were *on the way* to becoming diabetic.

This chronic, degenerative disease is being diagnosed with increasing frequency. Doctor's offices are overcrowded today with diabetic patients who have been treated with insulin and oral drugs over a period of ten to twenty years. Unfortunately, these very patients have advanced stages of blindness, kidney failure, coronary heart disease, and assorted nerve damage. Drugs by themselves are not the answer.

Early diagnosis of diabetes is important because it is a progressive disease with eventual disabling or lethal effects. But early diagnosis is extremely difficult. The disease can exist for twenty years without symptoms. The biochemical disturbance it creates, however, can do vast damage.

The most common form of the disease can be prevented.
Diabetes exists in two forms: juvenile and adult. The juvenile type is caused by a lack of insulin production in the islands of Langerhans in the pancreas. This lack can be due to tumors of the pancreas, surgery, or disease.

The most common form, by far, however, is adult or maturity-onset diabetes. Nearly eighty percent of all diabetic cases are of this type. The disease is seldom diagnosed until a patient is past thirty-five, so it is working its degenerative changes long before being detected.

These changes increase in severity and frequency with time. Among people aged forty-five to sixty-four, diabetes assumes ever-greater importance as a serious medical and health problem. The disease reaches its peak incidence at these ages, and mortality rates show a marked increase.

A national health survey indicates that diabetes is ten times more prevalent in those forty-five years old and older than among those under forty-five. Fifty percent of the known diabetics are within the forty-five-to-sixty-four age group when diagnosed. Thus, early diagnosis of diabetes would be of tremendous importance in the prevention of the degenerative damage it produces.

The diagnosis of hypoglycemia is significant in the prevention of diabetes, especially the adult form. If an individual is suffering from hypoglycemia now, he is a potential diabetic. Recognition and proper treatment of hypoglycemic patients means early treatment for potential diabetics and cardiovascular-diseased patients. That is why an effective program to prevent diabetes is predicated on an effective program to prevent and treat hypoglycemia.

The conclusion that hypoglycemia precedes diabetes is not new. Dr. Harris suggested the correlation while studying hypoglycemia in the thirties. Hypoglycemia itself has never received the recognition diabetes has; diabetes has been known to medical researchers for thirty-five hundred years, but hypoglycemia, as noted earlier, was not discovered until this century.

Diabetes cannot be corrected by insulin alone. Despite this fact, some diabetics are still told they can eat anything they want because more insulin can be administered if sugar appears in the urine. Unfortunately, insulin does *not* protect against many of the associated ailments of diabetes, but eating correctly can.

Insulin seems less of an omniscient power when we consider the fact that researchers discovered diabetes mellitus victims who secreted enough insulin to make them normal, yet still exhibited sugar in their urine: they continued to exhibit diabetic signs. In some cases, insulin levels were above normal, not because insulin was oversecreted but, rather, because it was underremoved; the body couldn't use it.

Suddenly, doubts arose as to the specific correlation between sugar levels and insulin. ". . . An orderly relationship between glucose and insulin concentrations [is] not apparent," noted Dr. Robert Metz, director of the Mason Clinic Research Center, after he examined a series of studies on twenty-seven research patients in 1972.

The primary action of insulin is to affect the transport of sugar into the cells. The hormone itself is affected by the changes in cellular activity induced by the cell's nutrient intake; the action of insulin is affected by cellular change due to the lack of nutrients. Thus, both diabetes and hypoglycemia can be the result of several factors, including nutrient intake and the manner in which the cells handle the intake.

Proper nutrition can prevent the ravages of either form of diabetes. The disease results from a disturbed metabolism that is directly related to inherited genetic weakness and malnutrition. The liver, among other organs, is involved in this disturbance. In diabetes, the liver's function of storing blood sugar as glycogen and releasing it as glucose is affected, and the organ may release more sugar into the bloodstream than the normal insulin supply can handle.

Dr. John Yudkin suggests that in countries in which sugar is used most (the industrialized nations), diabetes is also most prevalent. Other investigators have found cases in India and Africa in which members of the same family or tribe have moved into high-quantity sugar-eating areas. Those who remained at home, who never ate sugar, had virtually no diabetes, but the disease was prevalent among their urban cousins.

Sugar, the villain of malnutrition, weakens the body's resources enough to allow the genetic weakness to assert itself. And since it has no nutrients itself, it must rob other foods or the body's depleted reserves to use itself.

The cycle of diabetes is the same as that of hypoglycemia. Even the signs and symptoms—excessive thirst and water consumption, increased frequency of urination, excessive appetite, general weakness, itching of the skin, constipation, drowsiness, blurred vision, impotence, muscular pains—are similar to those associated with hypoglycemia.

Because hypoglycemia and diabetes are both metabolic abnormalities, they may often appear together, although they are literal opposites. In my own practice, I have seen hundreds of cases in which patients have been diagnosed as diabetics after they had taken a two-hour glucose test. Their glucose levels rise above normal immediately after glucose is administered. But *these same patients* will often exhibit a sudden and drastic drop in their blood-sugar level after the second or third hour. They "become" hypoglycemic. They are diabetics with hypoglycemic episodes.

Whether the physician is dealing with a diabetic or a hypoglycemic, he is actually trying to balance a metabolic abnormality. The body is neither receiving the correct nutrients for growth and repair, nor is it effectively using the nutrients it does receive.

By the time maturity-onset diabetes show itself, it is too late. Insulin and strict nutritional guidelines will control it—but why not *prevent* it before insulin is required? If the potential of the disease is recognized early, perhaps when its victims are first exhibiting mild hypoglycemic symptoms, we will have won a decisive battle in the war against diabetes.

Heart disease kills more than one million Americans annually. Many past victims of heart disease could have been saved or at least have lived longer if they had heeded a few simple nutrition-wise rules. Future deaths can be *prevented* if we begin to fight heart disease with a really effective weapon.

Prevention starts before birth, not when the initial terrible chest pains of coronary heart disease set in. The forces of prevention begin their work in the womb, where a child's first stages of life are supported by the vital nutrients contained in his mother's diet. Prevention will continue its work if the growing child is given all the nutrients he needs for his body to function at peak efficiency. With this kind of protection, his body chemistry will be kept in balance, and the fatty sludge found in arteries of heart victims, will never form. This child will not be another victim of what the late heart specialist Dr. Paul Dudley White called "one of the largest epidemics in medical history."

Dr. White's statement is not an exaggeration. Heart disease in the United States *is* an epidemic. Heart researcher Ancel Keys writes: "[In the United States] the question is not who has [heart disease], but rather who has more and who has less."

- Heart disease is the largest killer in the nation, accounting for fifty-three percent of all deaths.
- One of every two men over forty years old will die of coronary heart disease.
- The heart disease death rate has increased thirty-one percent since 1931.

In spite of these statistics, only twenty-seven percent of Americans over fifty-five years of age have blood-cholesterol levels checked during physical examinations. Fewer are tested for hypoglycemia, although unstable blood sugar is the forerunner of artery disease. A Glasgow, Scotland, study indicated that men over fifty-five years old have the highest death rate from coronary heart disease.

But heart disease is no longer the bane of the middle-aged man alone. Nearly seventy percent of American men twenty to twenty-five years old are seriously affected.

Women have just as many heart attacks as men if their reproductive ability is disrupted because of menopause, surgery, disease, or obesity. Pathologists have found diseased hearts in teen-age children. *The primary stage of coronary disease has been discovered in three-day-old infants.* Nearly all of a group of children studied in one test had fatty deposits in their arteries by the age of fifteen.

". . . Coronary heart disease has an incubation period just as do the well-known childhood infectious diseases mumps [and] measles, . . ." wrote Captain George L. Calvy, director of the Medical Field Research Laboratory, Camp Lejeune, North Carolina. "In the case of coronary heart disease, the incubation period may be 10 to 20 years.

". . . Coronary heart disease may be detected during the incubation period in nearly all such individuals. Once detection is made, the possibility of early and effective prevention becomes a reality."

The problem is so widespread that physicians have put most of their effort into treating the twenty-eight million adults who already have or are believed to have heart disease. But prevention is still the best cure. "Current intensive efforts to provide therapy for persons who have already developed coronary heart disease will undoubtedly save lives," notes a 1967 American Heart Association statement for physicians. "However, in view of the natural history of this disease, it appears likely that its . . . mortality can be substantially reduced through education and management aimed at preventing or retarding the development of atherosclerosis and its . . . complications.

"Preventive measures," it adds, "should be initiated early in life to have the best chance of preventing or retarding coronary heart disease. For example, correction of established adverse eating or smoking habits, while evidently beneficial, is certainly of less value than if the improper practices were never begun." But we should not underestimate the power nutrition has of being able to correct, at least partially, any damage that has been done.

"[The chemical changes in the body that produce atherosclerosis] are frequently brought about by the life-span pattern of diet," write Drs. Louis N. Katz, Jeremiah J. Stamler and Ruth Pick. "They are by-products of a habitually unbalanced diet excessive in total calories, empty calories, total fats, saturated fats, cholesterol, refined carbohydrates, salt, and inadequate . . . in certain essential nutrients (vitamins, minerals, amino acids, and essential fatty acids) and in bulk. Empty calories are calories derived from processed, refined foods, high in energy value and low in essential nutrients—foods such as sugar, white flour breads and pastries, solid cooking and table fats. . . ."

Most heart attacks are caused by atherosclerosis. This is a disease caused by soft, fatty materials that form in the blood vessels. It was originally thought that arteriosclerosis, or hardening of the arteries, was the heart attack culprit, but it was later proved that soft, fatty deposits of spongy consistency—atherosclerosis—precede arteriosclerosis and are the real villains.

The arteries become brittle only after their elastic fibers are stretched because of these clogging deposits. At that point, calcium solidifies in the deposits, and it eventually forms a plaque-like substance. As the plaque grows, the area surrounding it may become ulcerated or begin to hemorrhage. The fatty deposits of the early stage of atherosclerosis can be absorbed by the body, and the arteries will heal. But it's unlikely that any healing will occur once the disease progresses to the calcified stage.

Plaque growth in the arteries surrounding the heart soon affects the muscular organ itself.

The heart is a four-chambered, tough, hollow muscle about the size of a fist. It's an electrically fired pump which alternately squeezes and relaxes to push blood continuously through a flexible, closed system of pipes (arteries and veins). It uses one-twentieth of the body's blood supply just to nourish itself.

The heart no longer receives the amount of blood it needs once coronary disease strikes. The plaque in the arteries begins to layer, protruding into the hollow space once reserved for the bloodstream. A coronary artery may close completely. While the heart can function on a reduced blood supply, it will begin to deteriorate, just as an automobile engine loses power when its fuel line becomes clogged. The process, in most cases, is gradual; symptoms appear one by one.

One of the first signs of coronary disease is angina, an excruciating pain that begins in the chest and radiates through the left arm and into the head. The partially blocked arteries cannot bring enough blood. The anginal pain is a cry for help.

Angina can continue for years. One day, however, its victim's pulse may become rapid and feeble. His chest will feel as if a belt were being strapped fast around it. He may break out in a cold sweat, become nauseated, and vomit. The anginal pain in his left arm will worsen. This is a heart attack.

The attack can occur in two ways: When the heart has been starved long enough, it may become so weak that it can no longer keep a proper beat; it goes into a wildly erratic, shallow rhythm called fibrillation. The fibrillating heart does not have the power to pump blood to the body.

An attack also may occur when plaque breaks off into the bloodstream, sending large pieces of hardened material through the arteries. This material can cause a stroke if it lodges in the brain, renal failure if it lodges in a kidney. If it catches in one of the coronary arteries, an area of the heart will lose its blood supply and die. Also, the plaque can promote blood clots, which can enlarge and block the flow of blood in an artery.

The heart attack's severity is determined by the size of the heart area left without sufficient blood supply. Smaller coronary arteries sometimes enlarge, enabling the blood to bypass the clogged section. But the heart can be weakened enough so that its muscular fiber can no longer keep its shape; it will expand like a balloon and burst. Death then is immediate. If just a small area is affected, scar tissue will form. The heart will be damaged but may continue to work.

Nutrition can reverse the ravages of atherosclerosis. The American Heart Association attributes atherosclerosis, and the heart attacks it causes, to diet, heredity, stress, personality, other diseases such as diabetes and obesity, cigarette smoking, high blood pressure, and lack of exercise. Diet stands above all as the leading element and, fortunately, it is also the cause most easily remedied.

A diet low in essential nutrients—vitamins, minerals, unsaturated fatty acids, and amino acids—can cause the fatty deposits of atherosclerosis. These deposits are composed mostly of cholesterol and triglycerides. An overabundance of these two elements in the bloodstream is related to atherosclerosis.

Cholesterol is an alcohol compound that is found in nearly all the body's cells. The body makes its own supply to regulate the passage of nutrients through cell membranes, to help in the digestive system, and to aid in hormone production. It is a fat made infamous by the American Heart Association as the probable cause of heart disease.

Triglyceride is a neutral fat (neutral because it was originally thought not to affect the body either positively or negatively). Its name is derived from the fact that it is a combination of three types of fatty acids. Most of the fat we eat is triglyceride, and it's the same as what the body stores under its skin for later conversion into energy.

Patients who suffer from atherosclerosis usually have high cholesterol and triglyceride levels. But a great debate rages today as to what *causes* them to rise. Is it fat consumption, sugar consumption, or both?

Dr. Ancel Keys found in 1953 that coronary disease was more prevalent in countries where much fat was eaten. Fat was then supposed to be the prime cause of atherosclerosis, and the American Heart Association still believes this to be true. More and more researchers, however, suggest that fat consumption is only a contributing factor, and that the processed carbohydrates—especially sugar—are the chief culprits in the premature degenerative arterial changes that lead to heart attacks and arterial problems.

I believe *sugar* is the primary cause of heart attacks, along with cholesterol and triglyceride. This nutritionless food lacks the elements to work the heart's "furnace." The imbalances it creates make the body break down fats poorly. Cholesterol and triglyceride deposits are not the cause but the result of the problem; these deposits will form in a body that is not metabolizing its food correctly. The body will handle both fats easily if it receives the nutrients it needs to remain on a harmonious metabolic level.

I am not alone in my assumptions.

"In recent years, the pendulum of opinion regarding . . . atherosclerosis has swung away from the mechanistic view that ingested fat and cholesterol merely find their way through the blood-stream to the arterial wall," Dr. Margaret J. Albrink writes. ". . . Growing evidence suggests that an important and perhaps basic defect is in the area of carbohydrate metabolism."

Dr. John Yudkin, the University of London physician who has studied sugar for more than twenty years, argues that sugar's role in causing atherosclerosis is "already more convincing than the vastly greater body of information that dietary fat is a major culprit."

International statistics show a closer relationship between the coronary death rate and sugar consumption than Dr. Keys's initial correlation between heart disease and fat consumption. Sugar has become a major food product only in the last one hundred years, and fat consumption in most affluent nations has remained relatively stable during that period.

Other researchers are finding Dr. Yudkin's sugar studies valid. Dr. Cohen, an Israeli researcher, compared Yemenites who had moved to Israel twenty years earlier with those newly arrived. The recent immigrants had been on a high-cholesterol diet of meat and butter but little sugar. Few developed coronary disease. The reverse was true for the older immigrants who had accepted the Israelis' high-sugar diet. This correlation holds true for every industrialized country; as sugar usage increases, so does the incidence of heart disease.

Dr. Yudkin concluded from his own studies that a person who eats more than four ounces of sugar a day "was perhaps five or more times as likely to develop [a heart attack] as one taking less than [two ounces] a day." In two of his studies, in which he compared a group of heart-attack victims with a healthy group, he discovered that the diseased group ate nearly twice as much sugar as the control group.

Dr. Yudkin hopes to stop heart disease through preventive rather than curative medicine. Nitroglycerin, a drug that slightly expands clogged arteries, allows millions of angina sufferers brief respite from terrible pain, but it does not prevent heart disease. Proper nutrition does, but it takes a conscientious effort on every individual's part to change his diet. A 1956 study of the American Medical Association reported: "[The American] diet is pernicious to the cardiovascular system not only because of its excess in calories, [fats] and cholesterol. . . . It tends to be . . . high in . . . 'empty calories,' . . . foods rich in energy but low in essential nutrients."

Sugar is richest in energy and lowest in nutrients. The first step in any dietary improvement, then, is elimination of sugar and the other sickness-breeding calories found in most of our bakery goods. Quality food should be eaten instead, so that the heart is supplied with the more than forty nutrients it needs to function properly.

Cholesterol is a necessary component of good nutrition. You needn't stop eating foods high in cholesterol if you follow a proper high-protein, low-carbohydrate regimen that includes all of the essential nutrients. Fat- or cholesterol-rich food is *necessary* for two reasons: the body cannot absorb vitamins A, D, E, and K without such products, and a total lack of fats in the diet triggers the body's own cholesterol-producing machinery to secrete more.

If we accept the fact that arterial degeneration is a tragic end result of metabolic dysequilibrium, then we can begin to end the rise in cardiovascular disease. We need to understand that unstable blood-sugar levels, starting with hypoglycemia, are an indication of heart-disease potential.

As many as fifty million Americans suffer from some type of allergy. The allergic patient is one of the most tormented in the medical world, and he may try anything to stop the symptoms of his particular nemesis.

Whether it be asthma or an allergic reaction to food, drink, drugs, smoke, chemical vapors, animal hairs, insect bites or stings, toothpastes, cosmetics, perfumes, shaving lotions, or, the most common of all, pollen, the disorder does not respond well to attempts at a cure or even temporary relief.

Allergic reactions were first recognized for what they were in 1906, by an Austrian physician, Clemens von Pirquet. In early allergy treatment, doctors noted that the best "cure" was avoidance. For example, the most effective solution for a pollen allergy is, simply, to avoid environments of high pollen count. The technique works only if the victim discovers exactly which types of pollen affect him. The three major kinds—trees, grasses, and weeds—may cause discomfort during the spring, summer, or fall. Ocean voyages or trips above the timberline, however, clearly are not possible for most, although such trips are successful. An air conditioner provides some respite indoors, but this interim kind of relief far from solves the basic problem. It's difficult to avoid completely the offending elements that leave victims with sneezes, coughs, nasal blockage, sore throats, constipation, hives, itchy eyes, stomachaches, headaches, dizziness, and even asthma.

One person's allergic reaction may be quite different from that of another, although each may have allergies generated by the same source. Each individual has his own chemical makeup and his own particular reaction. The key question remains, not as to the poisoning agent or allergen—which can be almost anything organic, living or inanimate—but as to why some elements poison one person and not another. What makes one individual overly sensitive to cold water and another allergic to goose feathers?

More and more investigators of allergies stress psychological factors. These researchers have long suspected that deep-seated emotional disturbances lie behind a vast number of the cases that come before them. Some psychiatrists have found a high correlation between allergies and emotional upset among children who have difficulties with their parents, especially their mothers.

Researchers also have found a high incidence of allergies among emotionally disturbed children in institutions for delinquents. This finding was reinforced by a report made during the First International Congress of Social Psychiatry, at which physicians spoke of cases in which food allergies lessened at the same time behavior improved.

Many doctors believe allergies are psychosomatic in nature, that is, they are caused by emotional problems and must therefore be resolved by psychotherapy. Emotional problems *do* cause physical stress, and in that respect they may shed some light on the true solution to the problem.

I believe allergies occur in those people whose systems, because of metabolic imbalances, do not have the capacity to cope with stress. Metabolic dysequilibrium is again the major factor, and the wheezes of asthmatics and the congestion of allergy victims are again the body's cries for help to shore up its nervous system with needed nutrients. A body that is unable to handle the stress in its environment because of combined nutritive and genetic elements will manifest this inability in a variety of ways. One way is through exaggerated sensitivity to nearly any substance or condition—pollen, lack of sleep, even a bee sting.

Since the mid-thirties, physicians have found that allergies tend to run in families. If one or both parents have allergies, their children are more likely to have them than children whose parents are allergy-free. The allergy need not be the same in terms of either the reaction itself or the allergen that causes it.

The heredity theory suggests that an individual's genetic makeup may have a chink in its chemical "armor" that weakens the body enough to allow an allergen to have its effect. The victim reacts too sensitively to substances which, in similar amounts, are virtually harmless to others.

An allergy will always be worse if the body is not capable of resisting the stress placed upon it. If nutrition is poor, the body's capabilities are necessarily weakened, regardless of the stress. While the forms an allergy takes can be incredibly diverse, *each* form is based on the inability of the body to resist stress.

Allergies and hypoglycemia. Allergy patients usually suffer from the traditional hypoglycemic symptoms: nervousness, exhaustion, apprehension, weakness, fatigue, depression, and insomnia. These symptoms are exceptionally strong after physical, emotional, or infectious stress, as they are in hypoglycemia.

Allergy victims often eat large amounts of refined sugar, as do hypoglycemics. Their blood-sugar levels are usually low; when low enough, researchers have discovered, their allergic reactions appear.

One of my patients, a teacher in Houston, suffered through years of aggravation and misery from chronic bouts with allergies. Several doctors had given her skin-patch tests to discover which substances she was allergic to, and each physician found a host of positive responses. All told her what she could and could not eat, but not one stopped her from eating the large amounts of candy and sweets she craved, and her allergic reactions worsened.

"I realized that I could not enjoy an alcoholic drink of any kind," she told me. "As much as I enjoy a glass of good wine, I was unable to tolerate it; allergy symptoms—sinus blockage—followed almost immediately. I would invariably put in a miserable night propped up on pillows hoping to get one nasal passage open for normal breathing."

Finally, after her worst hay fever bout in fifteen years, she completed a five-hour glucose tolerance test along with other blood and hormone studies. She was hypoglycemic.

It took several months to rebuild her body's depleted reserves, but she recovered. As her hypoglycemia disappeared, so did her chronic allergies. Therapeutic augmentation of vitamins and minerals evened her blood-sugar level so she no longer craved the sweets that had twisted her body's metabolism.

Allergists rarely use nutritional programs to fight allergies, but they do use hormonal drugs such as cortisone and adrenalin. Some have used them successfully, which is understandable, because these drugs raise blood-sugar levels—exactly the effect of a good diet.

Instead of learning to live with her allergies, as the teacher was once told to do, and finding temporary relief from allergy symptoms, it was possible to treat the actual problem directly. It was possible to compensate for her weak genetic structure and consequent metabolic dysequilibrium by improving her body chemistry through sensible eating and medication.

My findings correspond to those of a number of researchers who found that hypoglycemics who suffered from allergies lost them when the disease was alleviated.

More recent findings also point in this direction. A Massachusetts physician wrote in *Obesity and Bariatric Medicine:* "During a glucose tolerance test, I have frequently found the patient [to have] an itching skin or even hives, a runny nose [or] a headache. . . . All of these are quite common allergic symptoms. . . . I have done six-hour glucose tolerance tests on over 600 patients, and draw my conclusions out of this rather large population. I have also followed the technique of having the patient run in place for five minutes at either the third-and-a-half or the fourth hour. This markedly brings the symptoms out. Not only do we see the blood sugar plummet, . . . but we see the allergic reactions come to the fore. . . . Sometimes asthmatic attacks will occur in a person susceptible to asthma."

All asthmatics have low blood sugar. (But not all hypoglycemics are asthmatic or allergic.) *No* exceptions to this rule have yet been found in a number of highly controlled experiments. Dr. Harris discovered that when asthmatics were given glucose-tolerance tests, their blood-sugar levels dipped below normal in every case. Several hundred asthmatics have been tested since, and all showed positive results for hypoglycemia.

Bronchial asthma is probably the most extreme of all allergic reactions. It is one of the most common and most debilitating of upper-respiratory problems. This condition has affected man since he began to react to his environment. Indians of both Americas suffered through its choking spasms two thousand years ago. The Indians' curative approach wasn't much different from ours, but in their case nature provided the necessary barks and herbs to treat the problem. Remedies such as belladonna and cubeb (a spicy fruit of a shrub) are still used by the southwest American Indians; they roll these into cigarettes or smoke them in pipes for asthmatic relief.

Asthma differs from other allergic reactions only in severity. Where hay fever may produce coughs, sneezes, and nasal blockages often associated with colds, bronchial asthma, or, more specifically, the allergens that cause it, affect the small air passages in the lungs, the bronchi.

Asthmatics have been aided by drugs that raise the blood-sugar level and by glucose shots. The sudden rise in blood sugar supplies their systems with the needed boost, and their symptoms disappear. But, as noted earlier, when the hypoglycemic is given sugar for symptomatic relief, the relief is only temporary. The *true* result is not relief at all, but another hypoglycemic attack. The additional sugar only worsens the rampant metabolic imbalance. Give a sugar "cure" to an asthmatic, as some doctors do, and his response will mimic the hypoglycemic's—initial relief followed by further attacks. It isn't accurate to say that hypoglycemia causes asthma, since climatic and geographic factors must be taken into account. But it is true that hypoglycemia allows asthma to appear.

The fact that attacks are triggered by low blood-sugar levels also explains why many asthma victims suffer most in the early-morning hours. Some are awakened out of sound sleep and unable to breathe because the bronchi have been nearly sealed shut by asthmatic spasms. Early morning is the time when the body's blood-sugar reserves are at their lowest. While taking a six-hour glucose test, asthma victims often have attacks at the point when their blood-sugar levels are lowest. Every morning can be a "glucose-tolerance test" to an asthmatic.

Interestingly, no diabetic has been found to have asthma. There are cases recorded in which asthmatics have become diabetic, but when they did, their asthma disappeared. If the diabetic tendency was controlled, the asthma returned.

Researchers have found other converse relationships between diabetes and asthma. Asthmatics have too much potassium in their bloodstreams. Low amounts of that metal are characteristic of diabetics. Asthmatics are affected adversely when they eat large amounts of salt; salt often lessens the need for insulin among diabetics.

It's difficult to understand why more physicians haven't seized upon the correlation between the craving for sweets among hypoglycemics and among asthmatics. One of my patients, a prominent architect whose asthma steadily worsened over a period of twenty years, was virtually living on coffee, colas, candy, and high-starch food. He had been visiting an allergist for years without relief from drugs or desensitizing injections, and the allergist found no problems with his patient's diet. By the time I saw him, the architect was completely discouraged and told me he was "incurable." His face was colorless, his bearing listless.

I convinced him to stop drinking coffee and soda, both high in caffeine. The high-protein, low-fat, low-carbohydrate nutritional plan that works for hypoglycemics works as well for asthmatics. It worked for the architect, and his attacks lessened gradually. In a matter of months, *all allergic reactions* were gone.

The architect, however, had a mind of his own. He experimented to see for himself if it was his diet all along that triggered his attacks. He went back to his former eating habits, and his answer was immediate. The wheezing and congestion that ensued were enough to make him return to his new regimen.

Asthma and other allergies are related to chronic, degenerative diseases associated with metabolic dysequilibrium. Some attribute the rise in the number of allergy victims to the fact that we live in a more emotionally stressful environment. Others emphasize worsening environmental factors. Both play their part. But the real cause of the increase is the terrible nutritional habits of many Americans and the subsequent lack of defense it leaves in their genetic framework.

Today, malnutrition has been firmly linked to barrenness as well as to nearly every aspect of the reproductive cycle. Malnutrition plays an important role in the loss of male virility, as well as the loss of female fertility. It causes obstetrical problems in pregnant women, and it is blamed for congenital defects and mental retardation in the newborn.

No one knows the extent of the incidence of sterility in the United States. Although three million childless couples live in the country today, no statistics record whether they are voluntarily or involuntarily sterile. The number of involuntarily sterile couples is augmented, however, by the poor nutritional habits of our country's population. "In general, the more generous the diet, the higher the fertility; the more meager the diet, the lower the fertility," writes Dr. J. L. Rommer.

Virility in men also depends upon good food selection. A man's heightened awareness and correction of his poor eating habits can make him as virile and active after sixty as he was at thirty. It has been found that men who are still virile in their eighties and nineties subsist on diets rich in natural whole grains and other vital nutrients, and conspicuously lacking in refined sugar and white flour.

Also, good nutrition, along with exercise, reduces the chance of obesity, a major factor in the loss of virility and fertility in men and women respectively. Obese women tend to have irregular menstrual cycles, a sign of an imbalance in the reproductive glandular system and a cause of infertility.

A confirmed correlation between infertility and obesity was first discovered by animal husbandry researchers who found that highly prized, fattened animals are often sterile.

Weight loss has the effect of restoring fertility, especially when it occurs because sugar is eliminated from the diet. A British study found an increase in fertility among obese patients who lost weight by giving up sugar.

Men often cannot produce sperm when they suffer from severe vitamin-B-complex or vitamin E deficiencies; the supplementation of these vitamins has been found to correct this disorder. In addition, the prostate gland is partially responsible for the secretion of seminal fluid, and a deficiency in the mineral zinc can cause this gland to malfunction. (Only half the normal amount of zinc is found in the pancreas of diabetics, who are often sterile.)

Malnutrition acts upon the hormone estrogen to cause sterility in women. Estrogen stimulates the development of several sexual characteristics and, like any other hormone, its production depends upon nutrition. A deficiency develops when women are lacking in any one of the necessary vitamins, minerals, or amino acids needed to produce the hormone. Studies conducted in Leningrad and Rotterdam during World War II (when the number of malnourished rose drastically) found many more sterile women than before the war.

Middle-aged sterility is directly related to the deterioration of body chemistry. This deterioration is much like that of any chronic disease; it takes many years to evolve. Sterility in the middle years is partly due to the nutritional indiscretions during one's youthful years. A diet that will keep an individual alive, notes Dr. Roger J. Williams, is not necessarily a diet that will allow him to continue to reproduce.

Obstetrical problems among pregnant women. If the malnourished woman does conceive, her poor diet can cause her many more obstetrical complications than a woman who has eaten well.

It may cause death. Evidence exists that many of the 1,581 women who died giving birth in 1958 [1] were poorly nourished. Their bodies just could not take the stress of childbirth.

"This means not merely that [a woman's] nutritional welfare during pregnancy is the important requisite," says anthropologist Ashley Montagu, "but that her own nutrition during her whole life, including the period of her sojourn in her own mother's womb, shall have been adequate."

A woman not leading a nutritionally adequate life at best will create a barren environment for her child, and at worst will miscarry or give birth to a stillborn or premature baby. An estimated 400,000 miscarriages and 175,000 stillbirths occur each year in this country.

Many obstetricians are convinced of the importance of nutrition. "[Obstetrics] owes much to the science of nutrition and in time will probably owe more, since many disturbances of pregnancy are suspected of being dietary in origin," write obstetricians Nicholson J. Eastman of John Hopkins University and Louis M. Hellman of the State University of New York.

Most pregnant women eat only a fair diet. A Harvard study published in *The Journal of Nutrition* followed the pregnancies of 216 middle-class women. Only thirty ate what nutritionists consider a good or excellent diet, but just twenty ate what I consider enough protein. Thirty-three of the 216 babies born were stillborn, premature, lived for only a few days, or were physically deformed. Only one of the defective infants came from a mother who had eaten a balanced diet with plenty of protein.

More than twenty-two studies of poor-quality diets have confirmed the results of the Harvard experiment. No matter where the studies were done—Boston, Scotland, England, Burma, North Carolina—the results corresponded: poor nutrition led to premature babies, stillborn babies, or infant deaths. These same reports showed that malnourished women had more pregnancy complications. A six-year study in Oslo, Norway, for example, found that proper nutrition eased pregnancy-related problems such

---

[1] The latest year for which figures are available.

as anemia, cramps, numbness, constipation, neuralgic pains, low blood pressure, and edema (swelling).

Complications can arise for either the mother or the unborn child when even one vital nutrient in the proper quantity is missing. Some of the nutrients already accepted by most researchers as necessary during pregnancy are: most of the B-vitamins (thiamine, riboflavin, pyridoxine, pantothenic acid, biotin, folic acid, and B_{12}), vitamins C, K, A, and E, calcium, copper, phosphorus, iron, manganese, zinc, protein, and the many amino acids (tryptophan being especially important).

An early study by three University of Toronto physicians emphasized the fact that an expectant mother on a nutritious diet will improve her chances of having a strong, healthy child. In the study, 380 women were divided into three groups. The first group comprised low-income malnourished women who were given no nutrient supplementation. The second comprised members in the same income range, who received supplements of milk, eggs, oranges, tomatoes, cheese, wheat germ, and vitamin D. They were also given dietary information. The third was a higher income group, but these women also were given strict dietary recommendations. The second and third groups had significantly fewer miscarriages, premature births, stillborn babies, or infant deaths. The group given supplementation suffered *no* miscarriages, stillborns, or postnatal fatalities. Six percent of the low-income group without supplements had miscarriages; 8 percent had their babies prematurely; 3.4 percent gave birth to stillborn babies; and 2.5 percent of the infants died soon after birth.

Income level obviously has little to do with the rate of infant mortality. A Canadian study found that the native Indians of British Columbia had the lowest stillbirth rate in the country, although the group was one of the poorest. Most of the women had no medical assistance during pregnancy or birth. The answer, according to the investigator, appeared to be in their diet, mostly consisting of fish, fish eggs, and seaweed.

Congenital defects are also attributed to malnutrition. The infant death rate is "not the most important part of the picture . . ." writes Yale physician Edward S. Quilligan. "The submerged portion of the iceberg . . . is those individuals who do not die at birth but who . . . are never able to achieve their full potential as productive citizens. We have no idea of the magnitude of this problem."

Poorly nourished women give birth to more congenitally deformed and mentally retarded babies than do the well-nourished.

"[Congenital disease] is a relatively rapidly growing part of our burden in the practice of medicine," Dr. James L. Wilson of the Michigan Medical Center told an International Conference on Congenital Malformations. "In almost any part of our hospital ward for infants, almost 50 percent of the babies are there because of congenital [problems], and if we take the wards in the big university hospitals, the great referral centers, it can go up to 90 percent. . . ." Congenital deformities kill ten times as many children as those killed from the five leading contagious diseases. These figures *do not include* congenital diseases that may not appear until years after birth.

Research with animals has proven that nutrient deficiencies cause congenital defects. When rats were fed a diet deficient in pantothenic acid, for instance, over half the offspring born alive were deformed. Sows were fed a vitamin-A-deficient diet that was otherwise nutritious; every animal in the litters was born without eyeballs. Cleft palate, cleft lips, and extra ears also were prevalent. The control group, given a full complement of vitamins, had no abnormalities.

A report in the *Anatomical Record* related that when the vitamin folic acid was withdrawn from the diet of mother rats after the first eleven days of pregnancy, all but five percent of the offspring were born with a wide variety of defects. Yet pregnant women are often found to be deficient in folic acid. In one study, 55 of 250 pregnant women lacked enough of this vitamin. The investigator, in addition, found that pregnant women needed four times more folic acid than nonpregnant women.

A study by Dr. E. V. Shute, a noted nutritionist, related birth defects to a nutritional deficiency in fathers. A group of males who had already fathered congenitally defective children were given large doses of vitamin E before further conception. Only two of seventeen births that followed resulted in children with congenital defects.

In the early sixties, hundreds of pregnant West German women took a drug called Thalidomide. The tragic deformities of their babies, although caused by the ingestion of the drug, were actually the direct result of nutritional deficiencies. Studies completed since the tragedy show that Thalidomide interfered with the ability of the fetus to absorb nutrients from its mother; riboflavin, niacinamide, and perhaps panthothenic acid were prevented from reaching the fetus at a time when it needed these nutrients for limb development.

An infant born from a nutrient-deficient mother may be affected mentally as well as physically. As noted above, women who eat poorly often give birth to premature babies. Many of these infants tend to develop more slowly and to lack the potential of a full-gestation child. Katrina de Hirsch, director of the Pediatric Language Disorder Clinic of the Columbia-Presbyterian Medical Center in New York and a leading researcher into reading problems, found in a study of first- and second-graders that children born after a normal nine-month pregnancy were significantly ahead, in reading and writing, of children born prematurely. Other research has revealed: premature children in a poor environment have a lower IQ than full-term children in the same environment, and prematurely born children are more vunerable to neurological impairments and the generally harmful effects of poverty than are children carried for nine months.

A Guatemalan physician, Dr. Joaquin Carvioto, in a speech before the Association Symposium of the American Public Health Association, said: ". . . Efforts to reduce the incidence of mental retardation caused by premature birth and complications associated with childbearing include programs geared to improving the dietary habits of all women of child-bearing age and to providing nutritional supervision early in pregnancy."

The brain of a fetus or newborn child can be affected by malnutrition in a number of ways. As a most extreme example, nutritional deficiency in the mother will cause cretinism, a defect in which the infant's brain is permanently stunted.

As early as 1929, two American physicians reported in the *Journal of the American Medical Association* that breast-fed babies showed intelligence superior to those who were bottle-fed. Dr. D. B. Coursin wrote in *Nutrition Review* that chronic malnutrition caused significantly poorer response to central nervous system tests.

Dr. Carvioto's Guatemalan study found that the use of an American diet high in carbohydrates and low in protein caused low IQ scores. But the Guatemalan study is not alone in tying mental retardation to a diet also found to cause hypoglycemia. Three physicians at the University of Illinois College of Medicine suggest that hypoglycemia may be the reason why, in identical twins, one twin is sometimes stronger both mentally and physically than the other. The stronger may have had access to a higher nutritional level, while the other received less nourishment and therefore developed an imbalance in his sugar-regulatory system.

Ten separate studies have related mongoloidism to diet, but Dr. Gretchen H. Runge of the Austin State School in Texas found a specific correlation between the disease and hypoglycemia. She administered a glucose test to mongoloids. The glucose level dropped severely after sugar was eaten, as it would in a hypoglycemic.

Just as a child's body continues to grow after he is born, his brain also will continue to develop unless something prevents it. Environmental factors play a large part in his development, of course, but all the learning experiences available will not help if he is undernourished. In 1963, two American doctors found that a group of undernourished children differed by an average of 22.6 points in IQ from another group of well-nourished children who were as similar as possible in every other way.

Researchers have investigated a host of foods and nutrients, such as ascorbic acid and nicotinic acid, for use in mental improvement. So far they have found significant mental improvement with a high-protein, low-carbohydrate diet, supplementation of vitamins C and the B-complex, glutamic acid, lecithin and thiamine together, vitamin E, and ribonucleic acid.

The need for proper nutrition, complete with *every* necessary vitamin, mineral, amino acid, and protein, is vital for the good health of both mother and baby. It is the half of the nutrigenetic factor that can be changed, inherited genetic weaknesses having yet to be controlled by science. Mother *and* father must provide themselves and their children with the best possible nutrition, if they are to function at their maximum genetic capability.

"In an increasingly complicated world of sophisticated technology in which even a mild reduction in mental performance may be a serious handicap," says Dr. Carvioto, "the possible effect of early malnutrition on mental capacity and personality development should be a major consideration."

Hypoglycemia and Related Mental Disorders

8

"I am firmly convinced that one day all these [mental] disturbances we are trying to understand will be treated by . . . hormones or similar substances," said Dr. Sigmund Freud in 1927. When Freud made that statement, he was not refuting psychotherapy, the treatment he created. He understood better than anyone at the time the questions psychotherapy could not answer, and guessed that at least some of those answers would have to come from other directions. He was looking ahead to the areas of knowledge medicine would someday have at its command in the battle against mental and nervous disorders.

Freud clearly regarded biochemistry as the ultimate answer to diseases of the mind. But could even he have imagined that such conditions as schizophrenia, depression, anxiety, aggression, and suicidal tendencies could be dealt with successfully by using the simplest form of biochemical medicine—good nutrition? Or could he have considered that if metabolic equilibrium, or balanced body chemistry, could be restored through nutritional planning, many of the characteristics and problems considered to be totally psychological in origin would vanish?

A growing number of psychiatrists and researchers find it reasonable to believe that if good nutrition improves *physical* health, it may also improve *mental* health.

They agree, conversely, that malnutrition may be an important factor in making mental illness one of the nation's most prevalent diseases.

The correlation between nutritional deficiencies and emotional disorders is far from being universally accepted today. Yet science has come a long way from the stubborn refusal of previous eras to accept the *possibility* that mental illness could be caused by poor eating. It took physicians almost two hundred years to be convinced that pellagra was a food-deficiency disease. It took them another twenty to believe the same about beriberi. Today, more and more practicing physicians and researchers are listening to the echo of Freud's original statements.

"Whatever behavioral process takes place, . . . it is our belief that there necessarily must be concomitant or correlative biochemical reactions," writes one research group. "We cannot conceive of even a thought occurring without its counterpart of biochemical and physiological events.

". . . It should be clear that general biochemical principles which are applicable to the liver and lungs are . . . equally applicable to the brain."

Dr. Linus Pauling, the Nobel Prize-winning biochemist, wrote in *Science,* "The proper functioning of the brain is known to require the presence . . . of many different substances." Dr. Pauling has argued vehemently against psychotherapy as the only source of treatment for the mentally ill. In 1968, he coined the phrase *orthomolecular psychiatry,* which he defined as a treatment for mental illness that supplies the best "environment" for the brain's biochemical processes. A mentally ill patient might best be treated, he suggests, by first providing him—his brain—with the proper amounts of the vital nutrients he lacks because of malnutrition. The "proper" amount, he noted, will differ from patient to patient, because no two people are exactly alike.

Dr. Pauling's theories fanned the flame of controversy that rose from Freud's original work. Dr. Abram Hoffer, director of psychiatric research of the Department of Public Health in Saskatchewan, Canada, was one of those who found little success treating schizophrenics with psychotherapy and shock treatment. Because he is a biochemist as well as a psychiatrist, he was drawn toward orthomolecular psychiatry well before Pauling coined the term. After more than twenty years of work using biochemical techniques, and psychotherapy when needed, Dr. Hoffer told *Medical Counterpoint* in December 1972: ". . . Orthomolecular [psychiatry] will double or triple the number of [schizophrenic] patients made well [and] markedly decrease the relapse rate."

An American physician watched six hundred mentally ill patients lose their symptoms through nutritional supplementation and wrote: ". . . After seeing all those nervous ruins regain health, I do not think it is necessary for anybody to learn to live with his nerves."

"It . . . seems that the biochemical aspects . . . of the mind have become clear enough that formal philosophy must take official recognition of them if it wishes to portray a comprehensive and true picture of men and the world," writes Dr. D. W. Woolley of Rockefeller University. "Formal philosophers cannot continue to remain aloof from the laboratory. If they do, the full nature of consciousness may escape them."

Freud himself insisted that his theories be taken scientifically, not dogmatically. They should be challenged, tested. "One might ask me whether and how far I am convinced of the correctness of the assumptions here developed," he wrote. ". . . I am neither myself convinced nor do I ask that others shall believe them; or better stated, I don't know how far I believe them."

Most psychotherapists today rely solely on theories of Freudian analysis, in spite of Freud's own doubts and his speculation about the need for order within all body systems. Dr. Edward R. Pickney, a California physician, writes, "Biological psychiatry is rapidly achieving scientific proof that . . . contradicts the Freudian concepts of all mental illness being the results of infantile sexual trauma." He adds, "I do not know of a single case where a psychoanalyst, even one with a medical degree, perform(s) a comprehensive physical examination before commencing analytic treatment."

Many cases of mental disease can be eliminated through the control of hypoglycemia. One out of every ten Americans has a mental illness severe enough to require psychiatric treatment. Half are under twenty-five. The Joint Commission on Mental Health of Children estimates that many children—twenty-six percent in some poverty areas—demonstrate "crippled . . . emotional development by the age of four."

Biochemically minded scientists are searching for new methods to combat this critical problem. Those who believe nutrition is a factor in mental disease have found links between blood-sugar deficiency, hypoglycemia, and some mental disorders.

One such investigator, Cincinnati psychiatrist Dr. Harry Salzer, became curious about hypoglycemia in 1953. After investigating the disease for nearly ten years, he wrote, "It is my belief that . . . hypoglycemia is one of the most common causes of neuropsychiatric illness, [and that hypoglycemia] has been caused by changes in human dietary habits."

"Hypoglycemia . . . should be kept in mind constantly by all physicians, particularly those doing neuropsychiatric work," reports *Oxford Looseleaf Medicine,* a medical encyclopedia. "The presence of hypoglycemia may suggest some brain disease, . . . vascular accident [stroke], . . . epilepsy, acute alcoholism, amnesia [or] hysteria. . . . For these reasons, . . . patients with hypoglycemia frequently are referred to neurological or psychiatric clinics."

Hypoglycemia attacks the areas of the body that need glucose the most. The central nervous system, which, as noted earlier, does not store glucose but needs more of it than any other part of the body, is most susceptible.

The brain, the key part of the central nervous system, is the first to feel the deficiency when the blood-sugar level is low. That is why doctors can be deceived into believing that the illness of their hypoglycemia patients is the result of anything from psychosis to fatigue to hypochondria.

Suicide, now the eleventh leading cause of death in the United

States, kills more than 21,000 people each year. An estimated 400,000 more Americans are believed to attempt it annually. In the last decade, suicide rates in the fifteen- to twenty-four-year-old age group increased sixty-seven percent. Just how many were caused by hypoglycemia, a known cause of depression?

More than eight thousand murders are committed annually in the nation. Most of them occur during intense family arguments or moments of stress, and they usually appear to have little rational motive. They are often committed by men or women with no previous criminal records. Might their behavior be affected, at least in part, by a severe low-blood-sugar attack?

Rob, twenty-three, tried to strangle his mother after a family argument. He was diagnosed as depressed, suicidal, and hostile. He underwent a series of six shock-therapy treatments after his murder attempt. Nine months later, his symptoms returned. Dr. Harry Salzer then became Rob's physician. He ordered a test for hypoglycemia and closely monitored Rob's nutritional habits.

The test showed the familiar hill-and-valley pattern of a hypoglycemic's blood-sugar level. Rob's diet was typical of undiagnosed hypoglycemics. He existed on coffee and caffeinated sodas, loved chocolate and anything else sweet, and filled himself with foods high in carbohydrates but low in protein. The sweets and caffeine weakened his sugar-regulatory system enough to make him hypoglycemic.

Rob returned to Dr. Salzer's office a month after he was placed on a new eating program high in protein and low in carbohydrates. "I am better than I have been in years," he said. He still is.

Dr. Salzer found a hypoglycemic condition "present and unrecognized in hundreds of [psychiatric] patients," and reported this to the American Medical Association in 1957. Most of Dr. Salzer's 300 hypoglycemia patients showed symptoms that doctors who are unaware of the manifestations of low blood sugar would consider to be psychotic: 180 reported symptoms of depression; 150 suffered from insomnia; 150 were chronically anxious; 135 were constantly irritable; 96 had crying spells; 93 reported various types of phobias; 90 said they lacked the ability to concentrate; 78 reported periods of forgetfulness or confusion; 66 showed unsocial or antisocial behavior; 60 complained of chronic restlessness; 36 evidenced psychotic episodes; 30 patients complained of suicidal urges.

Dr. E. M. Abrahamson, long an investigator of low blood sugar, discovered hypoglycemia in most of 220 neurotic patients he tested. These patients were placed on a low-carbohydrate, high-protein regimen. "Not only did they improve with respect to their physical complaints, but their purely psychic symptoms waned and abated," Dr. Abrahamson wrote in *Body, Mind and Sugar*. "They became so much more receptive to psychiatric persuasion that [psychotherapy] no longer had to fight against the usual resistance that neurotics display toward suggestion."

Real help for victims of schizophrenia. While men like Dr. Abrahamson and Dr. Salzer were discovering that hypoglycemia could cause neurosis, other nutritional investigators were tying low blood sugar and vitamin deficiencies to schizophrenia.

Of the 366,815 patients who are confined to U.S. mental hospitals, about half, the largest single group, are schizophrenics. Schizophrenia is a disorder characterized by the victim's loss of contact with his or her environment. Two million Americans will at some time in their lives feel its symptoms.

Only one-third of them will recover without aid. For the rest, results are dismal even with highly sophisticated professional help. A 1971 study states: "In the U.S., between 15 and 25 percent of all discharged patients will eventually be readmitted and receive continued care for a prolonged period of time. . . . Only 15 to 40 percent of schizophrenics living in the community achieve what might be termed an average level of adjustment."

Sharp battle lines concerning the causes of schizophrenia have been drawn between environmentalists and biochemists. For the environmentalists, schizophrenia is a disorientation of the mind brought about by environmental factors, that is, the victim's past and present living conditions. The biochemists argue that schizophrenia is closer to a deficiency disease or a malfunction of the body's chemical balance.

In the early fifties, evidence began to show that victims of pellagra, a disease caused by a lack of vitamin B_3 and protein, exhibited symptoms similar to those of schizophrenics. These symptoms were light-headedness, irritability, paranoia, unprovoked rage, and crying spells. Dr. Hoffer in Saskatchewan speculated that if pellagra symptoms were relieved by large doses of vitamins, specifically B_3 (niacin), perhaps the schizophrenic's comparable symptoms could also be reduced by the same treatment.

He began treating a young male student who was brought to his hospital in Weyburn, Saskatchewan, in 1952. The patient did not respond to shock therapy. He did not eat. He was incontinent. He was nearing death. A stomach pump was used to force ten grams of niacinamide (a niacin compound) and five grams of ascorbic acid (vitamin C) into him. The second day, he took the medicine himself. The third day, he sat up. After a month, he went home with vitamin C and niacin supplements and a high-protein, low-carbohydrate diet. He has not had a relapse.

Because my own work deals so much with low blood sugar, I see many persons who exhibit emotional symptoms. I've tested dozens of schizophrenics, and seventy-five percent of them had hypoglycemia. Jim, a bright student in his high school in a small west Texas town, had broken down at the end of his sophomore year in college. He was institutionalized and diagnosed as a schizophrenic by staff physicians.

Jim's family doctor visited regularly, but would not test the boy for low blood sugar. Jim remained hospitalized. He was brought home eventually, although he had not improved. He was unable to concentrate, and refused to participate in family functions. The family called me, and I asked their doctor to administer a glucose-tolerance test. The test showed that Jim was severely hypoglycemic, and he was immediately placed on a proper nutritional regimen, given supplemental injections of nutrients and continuing psychiatric care. He began to show improvement at once.

Dr. Hoffer named his treatment megavitamin therapy. He gives schizophrenics massive doses of niacinamide (up to 30 grams daily) and ascorbic acid (as much as 20 grams daily), as well as lesser doses of other nutrients. Megavitamin therapy, like Dr. Pauling's orthomolecular psychiatry, provides the body and its nervous system with the extra nutritional material it needs to make up for its deficiencies.

Nutrient therapy can lower suicide rates. Nearly six thousand schizophrenics kill themselves each year, a proportion that's a startling twenty-five times higher than any other single known cause among suicide victims. *There were no suicides in the 350 cases of schizophrenia Dr. Hoffer examined and treated over a ten-year period.*

Although Dr. Hoffer learned that megavitamin therapy worked, he didn't know why. He and his colleagues began to search for organic causes of schizophrenia.

They found that some schizophrenics have a chemical imbalance in their systems, the imbalance I term metabolic dysequilibrium. For some reason, these people use up excessive amounts of an enzyme the body needs for respiration, and when the body lacks this enzyme, Dr. Hoffer discovered, the adrenal glands produce a crystalline substance that acts as a hallucinogen.

This hallucinogen distorts the victim's perception and causes schizophrenic symptoms. Experiments revealed that vitamin C neutralized the hallucinogen and controlled the symptoms. Niacinamide helped the body build enough of the respiratory enzyme to correct the imbalance.

Subsequent studies confirmed this finding. In 1962, Dr. G. Milner, a psychiatrist at the Towers Hospital in Leicester, England, discovered that his schizophrenic patients were not only burning up quantities of the respiratory enzyme that Dr. Hoffer had found, but vast amounts of ascorbic acid as well—in some cases ten times more than normal. Dr. Milner concluded that low ascorbic-acid levels in the blood exaggerated a patient's existing condition. Large doses of vitamin C, Dr. Milner said, can improve a schizophrenic's condition to the point that he is able to return to a normal way of life.

Dr. Hoffer, Dr. Pauling, and Dr. Milner do not suggest that every case of schizophrenia can be laid to one cause and cured with one method. All three *do* believe that schizophrenia's present cure rate is tragically low because the treatment methods now widely used—psychotherapy, electrotherapy, and chemotherapy—simply are not adequate. Psychotherapy, at best, has only a forty percent success rate in the treatment of schizophrenia. In contrast, biologically oriented psychiatrists say their success rate is seventy-five percent.

As more researchers investigate the correlation between nutrition and good mental health, a remarkable number of vitamins, minerals, and amino acids have been shown to affect the central nervous system.

Studies have shown, for example: Patients who suffer from malnutrition exhibit depressive psychoses; patients who retain too much salt in their systems may go through similar states of psychotic depression; and amino-acid deprivation causes a marked increase in irritability levels. The B-vitamins play an important part in mental and nerve health. Thiamine (vitamin B_1) deficiency causes depression, irritability, confusion, and memory and concentration loss. It also creates a sensitivity to noise. Two 1967 British studies suggested that mental disease is also noted among people who lack the B-vitamin folic acid. In one study, forty-eight of fifty-nine elderly psychiatric patients were found to have below-average folic-acid levels. Also, loss of coordination caused by a disease called polyneuritis is attributed to a B-vitamin deficiency. Researchers can produce polyneuritis in animals by feeding them polished rice, a food lacking in B-vitamins.

Investigators have found that lack of biotin, a B-vitamin often called the growth vitamin, causes depression, confusion, and hallucinations. A deficiency of pantothenic acid, another B-vitamin, leads to nerve degeneration in test animals. Riboflavin (B_2) deficiency is tied to severe mental depression.

Two diseases that cause symptoms of mental disorder have been proved to be the result of nutrient deficiencies. Doctors *are* taught about two diseases, with symptoms of mental disorder, that researchers proved to be conditions of nutrient deficiency: pellagra and beriberi. These diseases affect both the body and the mind. Pellagra is principally a niacin-deficiency state, beriberi primarily a lack of thiamine. But neither disease can be cured with a single vitamin; each must be supplemented with riboflavin and vitamins A, B_6, and C. Pellagra patients have *died* with massive doses of niacin in them, while they were severely deficient in the other vitamins.

The discovery in 1912 that pellagra was a nutritional deficiency was one of the first instances in which a biochemical relationship to mental illness was drawn. ". . . When it became possible . . . to treat patients in mental hospitals in the southern United States with nicotinic acid and to find that a few of them became well (that is, the ones who owed their mental defect to unrecognized pellagra), a powerful argument was presented to some minds that other mental diseases of obscure causation might have a biochemical basis," wrote Rockefeller University's Dr. D. W. Woolley.

However, true to the tradition of conservatism in medicine, it took nearly two hundred years to achieve a genuine acceptance of the relationship of both pellagra and beriberi to nutrition.

Casal, a Spanish physician, described pellagra as early as 1735. His patients all exhibited the same mild, intermediate, and severe symptoms now listed as the four Ds—dermatitis, diarrhea, dementia, and death. Casal spent months observing Spain's peasants and their diets, and he correctly assumed that the disease was due to their negligent dietary habits. (Casal never named the condition. It took an Italian physician, Francisco Frapolli, to name it pellagra, or rough skin, after one of the disease's most distinctive symptoms.)

Casal's belief that pellagra had a dietary cause was backed by German naturalist and writer Johann Wolfgang Goethe, who wrote in 1786: "I believe that the cause of this sickly condition is found in the continued use of Turkish and heath corn." Like Casal, Milan's Dr. Giuseppe Cerri studied the impoverished in order to understand pellagra. He discovered in 1795 that local peasants were cured of the disease when put on the diets of the more well-to-do.

Through the nineteenth century, most doctors and patients thought the disease was caused by corn poisoning. Their argument reasoned that corn must be the villain because peasants ate corn products predominantly. The peasant, of course, had little chance to change his diet, and he continued to get pellagra, often developing the symptoms in a standard order—a red discoloration of the skin, digestive disturbances, and finally dementia which often began with nervousness, insomnia, memory loss, confusion, irritability, paranoia, hallucinations, anxiety, and depression. It ended in death.

American attention was focused on pellagra in the early twentieth century when it was found to affect many people of the South's low-income class. "In the insane asylums of the Southern states, over half of the inmates are there as the result of pellagra," Dr. D. T. Quigley, a researcher, wrote in 1943.

But twenty years earlier, Dr. C. Voegtlin initiated a U.S. study similar to that done by the Milanese doctor in the eighteenth century. Using pellagra patients in a Spartanburg, South Carolina, hospital, Dr. Boegtlin gave one group a diet that consisted primarily of corn products. The diet was similar to that eaten by the impoverished residents of the area. Another group was fed lesser amounts of corn pone and hominy, but more milk, eggs, and meat. The second group showed improvement, and many had complete remission. When they were put back on the original diet, their symptoms returned. The first group never improved.

A U.S. Public Health Service physician touring state mental asylums in the South had reached a similar conclusion in 1912. Dr. Joseph Goldberger noted that the medical and nursing staffs in the asylums, who ate balanced diets, did not develop pellagra. The patients, however, living on poor diets, did develop the disease.

Although evidence that pellagra was a deficiency disease had existed at that time for 175 years, orthodox medicine still believed it to be caused by infection, lack of good hygiene, even an adverse reaction to sunlight.

Dr. Goldberger, certain that the disease was not infectious, inoculated himself with the excreta, nasal mucous, and skin scrapings of pellagra patients. He remained healthy. He then went on to cause and cure pellagra in eleven Mississippi state prison inmates *solely* by altering their diets. At this point, most conservative physicians were persuaded. (But Dr. William Osler, justifiably one of the world's great physicians, died in 1919 still insisting the malady was an infection.)

Still, the substance that cured pellagra had not been isolated. It is here that pellagra and beriberi, also a mentally debilitating disease, are intertwined.

Most prevalent in eastern Asia, South America, and the Pacific islands, beriberi causes fatigue, loss of appetite and memory, irritability, emotional instability, confusion, gastric distress, abdominal pain, constipation, and heart irregularity. It took its toll among Dutch government and army personnel who managed vast holdings in the East Indies a hundred years ago. The Dutch government asked Christiaan Eijkman, a physician, to visit their colonies in 1886 to seek out beriberi's cause. It took him three years, but it might have taken longer if it were not for a touch of luck in the chicken coop.

Dr. Eijkman discovered that a disease similar to beriberi had broken out among his laboratory chickens. Checking his journal, he discovered that the disease occurred when the chickens ate the polished rice that was ordinarily fed to the soldiers. Beriberi among the chickens ended when a new army cook wouldn't "allow military rice to be taken for civilian chickens," and halted the dole. The fortunate chickens had to dine on their old unpolished rice.

Further tests on chickens and humans revealed that a diet consisting largely of polished rice consistently produced beriberi. Dr. Eijkman never did isolate a cure, but concluded that it was a substance in unpolished rice. His work, however, did lead to the discovery of thiamine and niacin, for which he was awarded the Nobel Prize in physiology and medicine in 1929.

By 1911, Casimir Funk, a Polish biochemist working in London, discovered four substances that he claimed were cures for pellagra, beriberi, rickets, and scurvy. All the substances, he said, were found in a good diet. He named these four substances "vitamines," and proved that pellagra and beriberi were inextricably related—both mental diseases that could be cured nutritionally.

Dr. Conrad Elvehjem of the University of Wisconsin further refined Funk's substances. He injected a purified chemical, which he called nicotinic acid, into a dog plagued with "black tongue," a canine form of pellagra. The animal recovered quickly. (Rather than have the public confuse nicotinic acid with nicotine in tobacco, a Yale researcher later changed the name to niacin— *ni*cotinic *ac*id vitam*in*.)

The case for pellagra as a nutritional deficiency disease had been proved by Dr. Goldberger, but it remained for Dr. Tom

Spies, a physician and nutrition pioneer, to show that the symptoms of *mental* confusion caused by pellagra began to appear far ahead of the earliest *physiological* signs. Looking back over his records, Dr. Spies found patients, facing him with pellagra, who had come to him earlier with a variety of emotional problems. He had found no trace of pellagra when he originally examined them and, therefore, hadn't considered it in his diagnosis. His pellagra patients, however, exhibited psychological signs years before the physical signs of the disease made themselves fully apparent.

Pellagra has not been eliminated in the United States. Thousands of its victims can be found in New York City and Los Angeles, the Appalachian mountains and the Louisiana bayous. These victims range from tired and irritable men and women, needlessly worried by "vague" but persistent symptoms, to men and women trying to cope with such problems as severe anxiety and depression. They have mild cases of the disease, and they can be cured with better eating habits and therapeutic nutrient augmentation in the form of vitamin and mineral supplements.

Behavioral disorders in young people are linked to hypoglycemia. Dr. Kenneth Moyer of Carnegie-Mellon University is one of the few researchers willing to take note of a relatively obscure fact: chemical imbalance, metabolic dysequilibrium, can and does have a sinister behavioral effect on the system of all humans, including young people. In fact, its effect on children is enough, when added to environmental factors, to cause antisocial behavior or other manifestations of mental disorder.

The Center for Studies of Crime and Delinquency in the National Institute of Mental Health is sponsoring research into the study of biological factors and their effects on violence. "The work has established that biological causes of violence are as important as the psychological ones—that no single discipline has a monopoly on the subject," says Dr. Saleem Shah, chief of the center.

The effect the nutrigenetic factor and hypoglycemia can have on the performance of children in school was noted in the previous chapter. The relationship can now be extended further: The nutrigenetic factor and subsequent hypoglycemia are part of the chain that causes juvenile delinquency. A child cannot have a well mind in a sick body. When an adolescent with a genetic weakness eats improperly, his *entire* body suffers, and a likelihood exists that the resulting imbalance will have its effect on the young adult's attitudes, temperament, and nervous system. Such changes have been noted by educators and law-enforcement agents who have studied problem children.

Most problem children have histories of school failure, and poor nutrition plays an integral part in that failure. "Delinquency begins with truancy," says Sergeant Joseph Phelan, a St. Louis juvenile-division police officer. Howard James, author of *Children in Trouble,* a book about the juvenile-justice system, says: "It is significant . . . that in at least 80 percent of all cases taken to [juvenile] court, one can find that a school problem was an important factor." Numerous studies bear out the findings of Phelan and James.

The delinquency problem is worsening at an incredibly rapid rate. Nearly half of all arrests for major crimes in the early seventies were of juveniles. Between 1960 and 1971, the crime rate for boys and girls under eighteen years of age jumped 124 percent. While most of these crimes were petty larceny, the FBI reports that from 1960 through 1970 police arrests of young people for violent acts rose 167 percent. In one year alone, 1970, that rate leaped 65 percent. The National Commission on the Causes and Prevention of Violence found a 300 percent increase in robberies over a ten-year period, 1958 through 1967. "We are now getting nine-year-old muggers," the police chief of Washington, D.C., told a reporter.

Most authorities argue that disinterest in school and subsequent delinquency occur because of a breakdown in the family unit or because of other disruptive environmental influences. Little or no thought has been given to a more tangible environmental factor, nutrition.

Malnutrition affects the metabolic processes responsible for a child's thinking and behavior. Ezra Benson, former Secretary of the U.S. Department of Agriculture, told a National Youth Power Congress audience: "Lack of knowledge about proper eating is a factor in the weakening of the American family life and the rise of juvenile delinquency."

Lack of nutritional knowledge in today's homes is the major cause of young people's mediocre diets. Many children are "sugarholics"; they crave sweets while skimping on more nutritious foods, and gulp sugar-loaded beverages in place of water and milk. Americans consumed about 184.2 bottles of soft drinks per person in 1955. By 1969, they were consuming 322 bottles, nearly one a day.

As noted previously, this kind of ersatz-food consumption is the quickest way to a chronic, degenerative disease, especially since the normal adolescent burns up nutrient reserves at a faster rate than at any other time in his or her life. During this period, the adolescent's genetic weaknesses, if not compensated for with good nutrition, will begin to surface and cause symptoms of metabolic dysequilibrium.

A Salvation Army study traced the eating habits of seventeen teen-age delinquents, all girls. They had been living on a diet of white bread, sweet jams, margarine, tea, and cheap canned or processed meat. When placed on well-balanced, nutritious programs, their behavior improved physically as well as emotionally. They were less belligerent, calmer, more willing to learn, less aggressive. Their new characteristics were "almost beyond recognition," better eating patterns having shielded them from the genetic weaknesses of their systems.

Antisocial or violent behavior doesn't strike suddenly. It begins early in a child's life and develops, if nothing is done to prevent it. Dr. Allan Cott, a New York psychiatrist, suggests that delinquency in a child may be the result of an inadequate diet on the part of his mother while pregnant with him years earlier.

There may be no problems at first, but by the time a child is in school and experiencing the challenges of education, the patterns of delinquency will begin to surface. Dr. Cott suggests that a bad beginning will proceed into an even worse development if the cycle is not broken. Many of these children, because of their poor prenatal environment, are or become hypoglycemic easily, and their diets must be regulated carefully. "The removal of offending foods from the diet of disturbed . . . children can result in dramatic improvement in behavior, attention span, and concentration," says Dr. Cott.

Judge Philip B. Gilliam of the Denver, Colorado, juvenile court astutely recognized the need for a nutritional approach in treating juvenile delinquency. During his thirty years on the bench he has heard over twenty-eight thousand criminal and juvenile cases.

"Deprivation of proper food is a very big element in causing many emotional and physical problems, including delinquency," he says. "Over the years, I have watched this very carefully. I find a great majority of the children coming to my attention are suffering from malnutrition. . . ."

Can a diet of candy, soda, overprocessed carbohydrates, and starchy food really be a causative factor in a child's mental disturbance?

The answer is yes, if we realize that stress exacerbates a metabolic dysequilibrium condition. The adolescent, especially, is under a high degree of stress. His social situation is one of constant flux and changing relationships. His mind and body are in turmoil as they adjust to their developing maturity. A well-balanced nutritional program will ordinarily provide enough fuel to compensate and absorb this strain and maintain the adolescent's metabolic balance.

But so few adolescents eat well. In the morning when their bodily needs for nutrition are greatest, some skip eating altogether, while others eat only a refined-carbohydrate snack, such as a doughnut or a few cookies. Lunch may be a sandwich consisting of a minimal amount of protein slapped between two pieces of refined white bread. As far as afternoon eating is concerned, J. I. Rodale in his book, *Natural Health, Sugar and the Criminal Mind,* says, "The after-school diet of snacks, potato chips, soft drinks and candy is one of the great enemies of youth today." Even if an adult of the family prepares a well-balanced, nutritious evening meal, the adolescent has a normal aversion to being a part of the family gathering at the table; he is likely to eat hurriedly and sparingly, and fill up on worthless snacks later in the evening.

I have seen remarkable recoveries among my own hypoglycemic adolescent patients when they're placed on a proper nutritional plan and are given vitamins, minerals, and other nutrient supplements. Incredible as it may seem, change can often be effected in as short a time as two weeks.

It may be easier to accept the contention that poor nutrition affects behavior if you consider the fact that other bodily disturbances of a biochemical nature affect behavior as well. Personality changes have been seen in youngsters after measles infections; behavior can be altered even by bouts with influenza. Yet most psychologists still don't look beyond the psychological and emotional factors.

Drug abuse among the young and low blood sugar. A great deal of attention has been focused on the young person and his use of drugs. A. W. Pezet, collaborator with Dr. Abrahamson in *Body, Mind and Sugar,* discovered that heroin addicts eat a great amount of sugar-sweet foods to reduce their urge for heroin. Dr. Abrahamson tested several addicts and found them to be hypoglycemic. Does the propensity for sweetness create an additional reason for adolescents, already suffering from low blood sugar, to experiment with drugs? We don't know, but it's certainly something to think about. Even if the connection is only a possibility, I feel that research in this area is of vital importance.

An incredible indifference underlies the study of drug abuse and criminal behavior in general. The United States spent $14 million in juvenile-crime research in 1970. It spent $18 million investigating tooth decay that year.

"What are we doing about today's children?" asks a Washington, D.C., social worker. "In Washington, we are doing just about the same as we were 30 years ago. . . . Day after day and year after year . . . we grind out services and treatment that have little or no relationship to our knowledge of the problems the treatment is supposed to solve."

The Joint Committee on Mental Health of Children, a nongovernmental research group, notes, "Each year, an increasing number of [children] are expelled from the community and confined in large state hospitals so understaffed that they have few, if any, professionals trained in child psychiatry and related disciplines. . . . Thousands upon thousands of elderly patients, now confined to the back wards of these state institutions, were first admitted as children 30, 40 and even 50 years ago. . . . One state estimates that one in every four children admitted to its mental hospitals can anticipate being . . . hospitalized for the next 50 years of life."

How many of these children have hypoglycemia? How many become addicted to drugs because of poor nutrition?

Tests for hypoglycemia must be made a requisite when a juvenile delinquent is arrested just as it should be made requisite for *every* person, child or adult, who is placed in a mental institution. Dr. Ben J. Sheppard, a Miami pediatrician specializing in neurological disorders and a former juvenile-court judge, argues for a host of tests. These "should include the child's whole social, educational and medical history. [They] should include [any evaluations] that might shed light on a possible organic reason for his or her behavioral problems."

If there is a chance that one adolescent can be led out of a delinquent's life, marred by crime, through critical nutritional correction, why is this avenue not investigated more thoughtfully?

Neither drug therapy nor institutional confinement offers solutions to mental disorders. The physician who prescribes only drugs for a mental patient who suffers from a nutrient deficiency may interfere with his patient's nutritional well-being, which is already in jeopardy. These drugs, whether they be tranquilizers, antidepressants, or anticonvulsants, increase the body's nutrient needs. They tend to deplete the body of needed fuel by slowing digestion and assimilation. The body must call upon its already limited fuel supply so the foreign elements, the drugs, can be used.

If a physician commits a hypoglycemic, pellagric, or other nutrient-deficient patient to a mental institution, he again worsens the condition. This "mental patient" needs good nutrition, and no mental institution I'm aware of supplies the planning needed for well-balanced meals or the between-meal feedings that will make the hypoglycemic or pellagra victim well.

The answer is an obvious and simple one: Give each incoming patient suspected of mental disorder a five- or six-hour glucose test. There is no way to know how many of the nation's institutionalized mental patients would be benefited by the hypoglycemic's diet—or how many would be freed of their conditions and their imprisonment. Sadly, no institution has ever initiated such a screening procedure.

Dr. Salzer put it succinctly: "A . . . glucose tolerance test and careful dietary history, particularly about the ingestion of starches, sweets, and intake of caffeine, are . . . indispensable for any patient presenting himself for neuropsychiatric examination. By making the diagnosis of . . . [hypoglycemia] and teaching patients what they should eat, many will be spared years of suffering, unnecessary operations, electro-shock therapy and the hazards inherent in taking sedatives, stimulants and tranquilizers."

"The future may teach us to exercise a direct influence, by means of particular chemical substances, upon the amounts of energy and their distribution in . . . the mind," Freud wrote. And "it may be that there are other undreamed-of possibilities of therapy."

Men like Hoffer, Spies, Salzer, Pauling, and Abrahamson have clearly shown us that some "undreamed-of possibilities" are at hand.

Alcoholism is one of the nation's most neglected and misunderstood health problems. Whether it be considered a mental or physical disorder (there is ample research supporting both), it's the fourth most common disease seen by physicians, coming after cardiovascular disease, cancer, and tuberculosis. One study of urban families indicated that as many as *forty percent* of the country's delinquent youth come from homes in which one or both parents are alcoholic.

An estimated $6 billion is lost annually by industry because of alcoholism's effects: absenteeism, loss of trained workers, inefficiency, medical care, and family support. Another $1 billion each year is spent in law enforcement concerned with the heavy drinker. About two million people are arrested each year for offenses that occurred while they were drunk. This represents nearly forty-five percent of all arrests. Federal government figures suggest that about fifty percent of the nation's convicted felons have an alcohol problem.

The pernicious effect of alcoholism or abusive drinking, however, takes place on the highway. By a conservative estimate, more than one million men, women, and children have died on American roads since the advent of the automobile. Nearly 103 million have been injured. *An American dies in an automobile accident every ten minutes, 6 every hour, 150 every day.* The financial cost in damages alone of these accidents has been estimated at *$180 billion.*

The National Highway Safety Bureau reports that while only four percent of American drivers are heavy drinkers, they account for at least half of the single-vehicle accidents in which someone is killed, and almost half of the fatal accidents involving more than one vehicle.

A University of Vermont study revealed that two-thirds of all traffic deaths in that state were caused by drinking drivers. A similar analysis by the California Department of Public Health found that seventy-four percent of the drivers killed in accidents had alcoholic levels high enough to be considered drunk by the National Safety Council's standards. Slightly more than half of New Jersey's drivers who died in auto accidents in 1972 had been drinking.

Hypoglycemia awareness can reduce the number of deaths on our highways. Not all drinking drivers are alcoholics, of course, but by reducing our country's incidence of alcoholism in some way, we can avoid a great number of traffic deaths. I believe there is a strong correlation between alcoholism and hypoglycemia. "One hundred percent of all alcoholics have [hypoglycemia]," says Dr. Abraham Hoffer in *Hope Giving Stories.*

The rising death toll of alcoholism either from cirrhosis of the liver or traffic deaths, is causing researchers to consider the condition more than they had previously. Many are still unable to find satisfactory answers to its causes.

While there is no universally accepted causal theory, there is no dearth of explanations. Most psychiatrists believe alcoholism is psychologically based. Physicians suggest physical reasons. Still other researchers say it's a combination. A poll of 781 physicians by a pharmaceutical firm reported that most felt alcoholism was a "symptom of underlying emotional problems." Other views, in descending order of popularity, were: a physiologic disease, a social problem, a behavior disorder, and a self-inflicted condition resulting from personal weakness.

The hypothesis that alcoholism is a sign of weakness may be closest to the truth. But it's not a mental failing as much as a biochemical weakness, in many cases, prompted by an imbalance in the blood-sugar level. Few physicians, however, treat alcoholism as a metabolic disease. Their attempts at psychological therapy seldom do much more than frustrate the alcoholic patient; those addicted to alcohol often have no serious emotional difficulties, but desire alcohol simply because they find it the easiest way to quell their body's demands for sugar.

No statistics indicate how many hypoglycemics become alcoholics, but as a result of my own dealings with thousands of hypoglycemia patients, I believe a definite correlation exists. Jack Martin had been an alcoholic for much of his adult life. Constant drinking had damaged his liver and he had gone through a bout with yellow jaundice. Jack finally defeated alcoholism with the help of Alcoholics Anonymous, but for the next six years he still seemed to be constantly hung over, although he had stopped drinking completely.

He awoke most mornings with terrible headaches and often found himself staggering about as if he were intoxicated. His pattern followed a similar one noted by Tampa physician Dr. Stephen Gyland, who found some of the six hundred hypoglycemics he studied to have been misdiagnosed as alcoholics. Their symptoms pointed to an uncontrollable lust for alcohol, which other physicians had assumed to be alcoholism. Treated with a high-protein, low-carbohydrate diet exclusive of sugar, their alcohol cravings lessened.

Jack Martin also was diagnosed as hypoglycemic after a diagnostic test, but he had not been told to stop eating sugar when he quit alcohol six years before. Alcoholics Anonymous found that most of its members could curb their desire for alcohol by eating large quantities of sweets, so Jack was encouraged to eat candy and other refined-sugar products, along with coffee heavily flavored with sugar. Unfortunately for Jack and many others, the sugar caused the same biochemical damage that the alcohol did when it was broken down into sugar by the body.

Jack withdrew from sugar altogether. His "hangover" symptoms vanished. He, like eight out of ten hypoglycemics, had an unquenchable sweet tooth.

Many hypoglycemics, like Ralph Miskif in Chapter Two, are only a step away from alcoholism. The hypoglycemic subconsciously will try to raise his blood-sugar level by eating foods high in carbohydrates, like refined sugar or alcohol. Unfortunately, the hypoglycemic who drinks massive quantities of alcohol will not only make his condition worse, but draw himself into alcoholism as his body demands more.

His already sensitive sugar-regulatory system will produce more insulin with each drink. The more he drinks, the lower the sugar level drops. He is trapped in a worsening cycle that will never be reversed by psychotherapy alone. Psychotherapy may help his problems, but only *after* he has been placed on a nutritious diet that levels his blood sugar.

But as I have stated before, blood-sugar tests are rarely taken. When they are, hypoglycemia is often looked upon as a *result* of alcoholism, not a cause. When Dr. Hoffer suggested that all alcoholics are hypoglycemic, he was alluding to the fact that if all alcoholics were not originally hypoglycemic, they developed it from drinking too much alcohol and not eating enough nutrient-filled foods.

Alcohol seeps through the stomach lining directly into the bloodstream, and isn't broken down until it reaches the liver. A well-functioning liver can handle the increased work load needed to detoxify alcohol, which acts like a poison in the body. But an alcoholic drinks much and eats little.

Alcohol can replace fats and carbohydrates as energy sources—an ounce of liquor has as many calories as a half pound of fish—but it totally lacks any of the nutrients the body needs to replenish itself. An alcoholic therefore can survive for days on liquor because of its energy supply, but his body will deteriorate at an increasing rate because it is not receiving vital nutrients. He becomes more and more malnourished by substituting alcohol calories for those he normally would get from wholesome foods.

The alcoholic's liver is placed under a great strain, having to work hard to break down alcohol but lacking the needed materials to carry on its work. It begins to store excess fat and becomes less able to do its real job of saving glycogen, the storage form of blood sugar (glucose). The victim cannot keep his blood-sugar level up. This is how alcoholics *become* hypoglycemic.

The idea that alcoholism may be caused by a poor diet is taking hold slowly among some researchers and physicians. Dr. Roger J. Williams, known internationally for his research into nutrition and who has long promoted deficiency disease as a cause of many illnesses, wrote: ". . . The uncontrolled craving for alcohol in certain individuals is a nutritional deficiency disease. . . . No one who follows good nutritional practices [could] ever become an alcoholic."

Dr. Williams found that some men or women are more likely to become alcoholics than others. They are of a biochemical type that has abnormally high nutrient requirements. Dr. Williams discovered that after high vitamin dosages, some alcoholics not only could refuse a drink, but could take one without having to have another. Dr. Aaron Prigot of the Harlem Hospital Center injected amino acids into alcoholics and prevented or reduced their delirium tremens during withdrawal.

Why some individuals have higher-than-normal requirements, and why they turn to alcohol as a result, is still a mystery. But once a person reaches an alcoholic state, his body fails to use properly what little nutrients it receives. Thiamine is absorbed poorly. The brain's ability to absorb its only fuel, glucose, is impaired because small arteries feeding blood to the brain become clogged. These arteries may eventually become so damaged that they cut off large portions of the brain's blood supply, resulting in the death of a great number of brain cells.

More research has to be done in hypoglycemia as a cause of alcoholism. Few researchers have continued Dr. Williams's and Dr. Gyland's work, even though it strongly suggests that low blood sugar may be a cause of chronic alcoholism.

Good nutrition and metabolic therapy will help any alcoholic, whether hypoglycemia is the cause or not. If the failing body chemistry of alcoholics can be metabolically balanced, if we utilize proper nutrition to restore their degenerative bodies, alcoholism, which is still increasing uncontrolled, can be beaten.

Obesity, Another Case of Malnutrition

9

Many Americans believe malnutrition is seen only in Asian or African lands, where children with bloated stomachs stare pitifully into cameras to elicit help from the world's richest country.

Starvation is, obviously, the severest form of malnutrition. But just as those children hide their starvation behind swollen, distended stomachs, many Americans hide their malnutrition behind flabby pot bellies. They are victims of a chronic, degenerative disease often called obesity, but better described as adipose disease.

Today, far more Americans are obese than ever before. The causes range from heredity and poor eating habits to our modern, sedentary way of life.

Heredity is a prime culprit. According to statistics, if one parent is obese, there's a forty percent possibility his children are likely to be; if both parents are obese, the likelihood rises to eighty percent. But if both parents are within normal weight parameters, there's only a six percent chance their offspring will be excessively overweight.

These statistics are a graphic representation of the genetic factor present in all of us. But as I've said before, this factor is only a part of the total picture; obesity is another chronic disease that is a product of genetic predisposition coupled with poor nutrition and the metabolic dysequilibrium it creates.

Of course, the condition is exaggerated by overeating and lack of exercise, but these are not the primary causes of the real *disease* of obesity, whose victims go through life grossly overweight and completely without hope, having tried every reducing method known to man.

The obese person is rarely told that he suffers from a chronic illness, that it is a degenerative or steadily worsening disease, or that his metabolism is out of order. Rather, he's victimized by a diet-crazed, scale-cult society, which surrounds and bombards him with repeated new diets that have as their sole objective weight loss instead of medical slenderizing and normalizing body chemistry.

A therapeutic plan provides help to improve health and to prevent further development of chronic illness. A "new diet" provides neither.

Diet should not be related to weight loss, but should be regarded as a method in which the body is given the fuel it needs to regulate metabolism and *burn fat properly*. If the obese person works toward restoring *health* to his or her body—the proper goal —the excess pounds will roll off in the process. Therapeutic nutrient augmentation assists the body's metabolic processes to burn off fat deposits and *prevent* new deposits from forming.

It's true that the reducing diets popular today, if adhered to, will result in weight loss. But not one of these diets includes enough proper nutrients to restore healthy metabolism and resolve an overweight problem *permanently*.

As long as our present emphasis on calorie reduction remains, the obese will continue the frustrating roller-coaster ride of repeated weight gain and loss. And appetite-depressant drugs are not the answer either; not only do these ignore the root of the problem, but they have the effect of slowing down the process of digestion. This *compounds* the problem, because sluggish digestion is one of the many conditions that results from metabolic imbalance and leads to obesity in the first place.

Americans today eat fewer total calories than their ancestors, but our less strenuous lives require fewer calories. As activity decreases, the desire for food intake normally lessens, but the reduction in eating is rarely proportionate. Thus, the most civilized countries suffer the most obesity. A British physiologist notes: "It is not generally realized how sedentary is the life led by most urban people. Even young military cadets spend 17¾ hours a day either prone, sitting or standing [still]. The daily physical activity of many thousands of light workers may be below the threshold needed for appetite to function normally. For this reason they may . . . become obese."

But the trend toward inactivity among Americans is not solely responsible for widespread obesity. Change in the American diet (toward less nutritious food) has developed simultaneously and as rapidly, and must bear part of the blame.

With technological developments in almost every field of production, from farming to steelmaking, came less physical labor and a dietary change that included more fats and processed carbohydrates and a rise in total calorie level. Americans forgot that there are two classifications of calories: "friendly" calories, which include those from protein, the complex carbohydrates in fruits and vegetables, and the unsaturated fatty acids; and "enemy" calories, derived from processed carbohydrates, found in refined sugar and flour products and saturated fatty acids.

Only a hundred years ago, Americans were more dependent on vegetables (fresh in summer, canned in winter) and whole-grain cereals. They looked more to poultry products for their protein. Their meat was leaner than today's specially fattened animals. It was impossible to keep meat, butter, and milk without refrigeration, so they ate less of these. There was no easy way to keep ice cream. With fewer candy counters and no vending machines, Americans made fewer stops for sodas and sweets.

". . . Not isolated men but whole populations have become relatively overweight . . ." in a food environment such as today's, says Dr. Lawrence E. Hinkle, Jr., of Cornell Medical College.

Twenty to twenty-five percent of the U.S. population today is overweight—fifty million people. However, all of these people are not obese. Some are overweight as the result of heavy bone structure or muscular development; the term obesity describes excessive body *fat* only. Thus, some people of normal weight, but of lighter-than-average bone and musculature, can be obese. But we will consider obese all people, regardless of body type, who are twenty pounds or more overweight.

About sixteen percent of the American population under thirty years old is obese. Twenty-five percent of all American men over thirty carry more than twenty extra pounds; the same holds true for forty percent of American women over forty years of age.

One of every seven American children and adolescents is obese —an astounding twelve million young people.

Although life-insurance studies show increases in the number of men and women who become overweight as they get older, the greatest increase appears among those in their young adult years, the twenties and thirties.

What do these young people have to look forward to? Their chances for an earlier-than-normal death increases by forty-two percent if they are only moderately obese, by seventy-nine percent if markedly so. Many will become diabetic and take on that disease's varied ills. Hypertension and the tagalong risks of heart attack and stroke closely follow obesity. Gall bladder, kidney and liver disease, digestive diseases, arthritis, respiratory ailments, and increased mortality from surgical complications all plague—and kill—the obese adult. One medical textbook overstated it somewhat: "The only cause of death that does not strike the obese more often than the lean population is suicide."

Despite these known correlations, obesity has been relatively little investigated. The American Academy of Pediatrics notes that "our ignorance concerning . . . obesity is remarkable."

Most doctors are unsure about obesity, its causes, its relief. They don't know how to identify obese patients with any preciseness. Most physicians use life-insurance company tables that list average weights related to height and body-frame size. These ideals are far too vague. How much weight is really too much? Is a football lineman, far above average weight because of muscular tissue, obese? Exactly where is the line dividing the overweight child from one who is obese—and, therefore, with the more serious problem?

Many doctors continue to stress obesity's psychological factors too strenuously. Their rationale seems to be that obesity is caused solely by overeating. Overeating, they reason, results from a loss of self-control which in turn is caused by a more serious emotional disorder. Such analysis leads to extraordinary despair among obese patients who actually are suffering from a physical disorder. These patients still are told they must learn to "control themselves." Some obesity *is* caused by neurosis, but the total is far less than those cases that result from physiological causes.

The loss of fat—all but impossible for many adults, and only fifteen percent successful among today's obese adolescents—is simply the reduction of a symptom of a particular metabolic difficulty. To treat a patient solely for weight reduction is like treating a tubercular patient for his fever. The physician may lower the fever with drugs, but the disease remains.

The doctor may be able to lower the patient's weight, but the underlying condition, the untreated metabolic imbalance, is always ready to recur. The patient remains untreated until he returns to the doctor with a more ostensibly threatening, but related, disease such as atherosclerosis or diabetes.

The doctor's recommended diet, usually one that cuts back on all calories without considering the *type of calorie,* is wrong. Protein calories must remain abundant, and saturated fat calories must be reduced, as should those of processed carbohydrates. Both the latter are major factors in the body's inability to burn fats properly.

If obesity is treated as a chronic, degenerative disease, its relationship to other degenerative diseases, such as heart disease and diabetes, becomes clearer.

Obesity in most cases is a long-term condition.

- At least half of all grossly obese adults were obese as youngsters.

- Eighty percent of all obese children become obese adults. The percentage is higher for girls.
- Cure of obesity on a long-term basis has been relatively unsuccessful.

It's clear that the best time to reach, and change, an obese individual is before he or she reaches the fourth or fifth grade. By high-school age, the metabolic dysequilibrium has already had too long a life, and obese young people by then are rocklike in their resistance to weight loss. The 1970 White House Conference on Food, Nutrition and Health reported that if an obese child reaches the age of twelve, "the odds against his being a normal-weight adult are 4 to 1; if weight reduction doesn't occur by the end of adolescence, the odds rise to 28 to 1."

The longer the body is chemically out of balance, the more deeply entrenched will be the effect upon its many systems. A car that burns its fuel improperly will build thicker and thicker carbon deposits. Also burning its fuel improperly, the imbalanced body builds its own clogging deposits of cholesterol and triglycerides (associated with heart disease), which may come to rest in the liver or on the walls of the arteries, and it also suffers from irregular blood-sugar levels (about eighty percent of the obese are either diabetic or hypoglycemic, or a combination of both).

Eating habits established in infancy can doom a child to a lifetime of fighting obesity. "The critical period seems to be the first year of life, . . ." says Dr. S. L. Hammar, pediatrician at Kauikeolani Children's Hospital, Honolulu. And "most [obese adolescents] will remain [obese] in spite of periodic attempts at weight control. Our present therapeutic approaches to the obesity problem produce notoriously poor results."

A Massachusetts study found that over ten percent of the children in one public-school district were obese. In an investigation in Cumberland, Maryland, 668 children between the ages of five and thirteen were examined. Ten percent were overweight in at least one of the three years in which the test was made. Of 3,508 students examined at the University of Chicago, nearly twenty-four percent of the women and twenty-nine percent of the men were considered obese. Researchers discovered that eighty-six percent of the men and eighty percent of the women who were overweight as children were still overweight as adults, in one follow-up examination of a group of adults who had been previously checked when they were elementary-school students in Hagerstown, Maryland.

The obese can suffer several possible physiological breakdowns. One of these can be an upset in the balance of the appetite-control mechanism in the hypothalamus, a gland in the base of the midbrain. One portion of the hypothalamus tells the body when to eat; another portion tells it when to stop. Normally, each counterbalances the other so well that only minute weight discrepancies develop.

Yet people have been known to eat food in huge quantities without quelling the hunger response. Others nearly starve to death because they have no urge to eat. These extremes illustrate severe malfunction of the gland.

But obesity can occur when even a slight malfunction develops; it takes only an infinitesimal imbalance to cause it. A one percent error in the mechanism can mean the gain of many pounds.

The healthier the hypothalamus, the greater its accuracy. Like any other gland, it is kept healthy through the nutrients it receives. The better an individual's nutritional habits, the better his appetite-control system will function. A positive cycle is created. If an individual's hypothalamus is prone to malfunction (the genetic factor), proper nutrition at least can make it work at its optimum efficiency.

Glucose levels, too, play a part in food intake. When glucose levels are high, hunger is absent. Once the level dips, a chemical reaction causes the stomach to contract and hunger pangs to develop. The obese don't always feel these pangs immediately. Conversely, they sometimes continue to eat once the levels have risen enough to still the pangs. Their controls are delayed. Although little work has been done on hormonal deficiencies and obesity, it seems that such correlations do exist. Between-meal and bedtime snacks of the kind recommended in Appendix II of this book can help to regulate these deficiencies.

Obesity is not overnutrition, as it is sometimes called.
". . . Many prosperous citizens of the Western world today dig their own graves through overeating," notes biologist Rene Dubos. Obese people do eat too much in *quantity,* but they are still malnourished because they select food of poor nutritional *quality;* they throw their control systems off by confining their diets to large amounts of processed carbohydrates and too-small amounts of vitamins, minerals, amino acids, and polyunsaturated fatty acids.

Low-calorie faddish diets further deplete the body's already exhausted nutrient reserves. Crash diets are particularly self-defeating because the rapid weight loss, without nutrient supplements, is apt to cause physical or emotional illness.

Weight loss, when properly attempted, however, is effective in lowering disease susceptibility. "The removal of [fat] can be of crucial importance in disorders of the circulatory and locomotor systems," says the U.S. Department of Health, Education and Welfare. "Obesity can contribute to their further [weakening] and appropriate weight reduction can greatly aid in their treatment. Among such conditions are angina pectoris, hypertension, congestive heart failure, . . . varicose veins, rupture of intervertebral discs, osteoarthritis, and many other varieties of bone or joint disease."

One medical-journal study found that seventy-five percent of middle-aged obese diabetics lost their glucose sensitivity completely after they reduced to their ideal weight. Half of the remaining participants improved.

No evidence exists, however, that cholesterol, once deposited in the arteries, can be removed by weight correction alone. But a properly balanced diet, with nutrient supplements, *can* prevent atherosclerosis by ridding the body of excessive cholesterol and keeping it from forming again.

Pharmaceutical companies, attracted to the lucrative field of weight reduction, have been creative in their efforts to find new and appropriate products. They have developed the appetite-depressing drugs that often have uncomfortable side effects, and the diuretics that wash out needed water-soluble vitamins and minerals, nutrients that the obese can scarcely afford to lose.

The best method for weight control is the prevention of weight gain altogether through exercise and proper nutrition. Exercise is an effective means of keeping fat from accumulating once one's metabolic dysequilibrium is corrected. In fact, exercise not only takes off weight, but it helps maintain a healthy metabolism. In any case, an appropriate nutritional and exercise plan should be designed by a nutritionally informed physician, not the dieter, although all dieters can benefit from the guidelines given in Chapter 5.

Good nutrition and exercise *cannot* be separated. With both, the body's organs receive more nutrients and more oxygen through increased circulation and the hypothalamus works in an optimum environment and at peak efficiency. Unfortunately, exercise is especially neglected by the obese, who rarely move more than they must.

The cycle of youthful obesity, depression, and withdrawal from social activity is hard to break, and is unlikely to be broken at all when it starts with the very young. Adipose disease almost assuredly will develop in those who have low exercise rates, because they tend to eat more to relieve the boredom of their sedentary lives. Exercise will firm and tone tissues and increase circulation, but it cannot do everything. It cannot overcome bad eating.

Ease into a vigorous exercise program. Exercise should not produce excess fatigue—the exhaustion that doesn't clear after a few minutes of rest—and no exercise plan should begin without a doctor's approval.

The best initial form of exercise is walking, beginning with a daily half mile. Gradually increase the pace until you can cover the distance in at least ten minutes. Then increase the distance. Jogging should be considered only after you've accumulated substantial reserves of energy through months of proper nutrition. Bicycle riding and swimming are also excellent forms of exercise. By increasing your energy output 500 calories a day, you can expend 3500 additional calories a week, an amount approximately equal to one pound of fat.

Every weight-correction program should be based on one principle: The body must release more energy than it receives. A diet recommended by a nutrition-wise physician *and* increased physical exercise will help you attain that end.

The following chart will help you plan a program for increasing your caloric output.

APPROXIMATE CALORIES USED PER HOUR ACCORDING TO BODY WEIGHT

ACTIVITY	100 lbs.	120 lbs.	140 lbs.	160 lbs.	180 lbs.	200 lbs.
Sleeping	45	60	91	112	144	170
Light exercise (Ironing, Cooking, Dusting)	95	132	182	240	297	370
Gardening	110	156	217	280	360	440
Walking slowly (2.6 mph)	130	186	252	336	423	520
Walking moderately fast (3.75 mph)	195	282	385	496	630	780
Walking downstairs	235	342	462	608	765	940
Heavy Exercise	290	420	574	744	945	1190
Swimming	325	468	637	832	1053	1300
Running (5.4 mph)	370	534	728	944	1197	1480
Walking upstairs	720	1032	1407	1840	2322	2870

Diagnosis and Treatment

10

Hypoglycemia is a common ailment, and although it is often associated with the signs of other chronic conditions, it is by no means the cause of every illness; in no way do I mean it to be all things to all people. With that made clear, I will commence with what is probably the most important and crucial aspect of this disease—its diagnosis.

If more doctors were aware of the ways and means of the diagnosis of low blood sugar, it would be recognized as a common ailment and receive the attention it deserves. It certainly demands more serious consideration than it received at a recent symposium I attended.

A lecturing psychiatrist there, in response to a suggestion that hypoglycemia might be the cause of some of his patients' fatigue, rather than depression and boredom, resented the thought that *anyone* should be treated for the disease. "These patients are even on special diets—and everyone knows that you get everything you need in today's food. They don't need special diets. All they need are tranquilizers and someone to talk to them about their problems." Another physician at the symposium said: "If anyone asks me about checking them for hypoglycemia, I tell them I'm not that kind of doctor."

These examples are small indications of orthodox medicine's large-scale, slow acceptance of relatively new or controversial medical tactics against disease. Dr. Emil Grubbe spent forty years arguing for X-ray therapy while cancer patients lived in pain and died without the treatment which is now generally accepted. Dr. Frederic Gibbs presented his electroencephalograph to the medical profession in 1934, but its value in helping to interpret the functions of the brain went unnoticed for years. Orthodox medicine still refuses to recognize the value of vitamin E in the treatment of cardiovascular disease and senility. Canadian physicians Evan and Wilfrid Shute, however, have documented thousands of cases that reveal unquestionable benefit for heart patients through vitamin E therapy.

It is much the same with hypoglycemia. The fact remains that the patient goes to the doctor to obtain relief from the symptoms he is suffering, and it is the physician's responsibility to be aware of diagnostic procedures. Because of hypoglycemia's medical unattractiveness, the *patient* may have to insist that the necessary diagnostic tool, a five- or six-hour glucose-tolerance test, be administered.

When a patient realizes that his symptoms are the result of a metabolic condition, especially after he has been told time and again that his troubles are psychological, his confidence and sense of competence are often restored. Proper diagnosis often overcomes the fear, confusion, and helplessness that plague the hypoglycemic.

The strictly psychological or psychiatric "diagnosis" of the mental and emotional symptoms of hypoglycemia virtually entraps the victim in an ever-widening cycle of misery and self-doubt. The hypoglycemic becomes entangled in his own behavioral symptoms, and develops a false perception of his disease. Something is wrong, he knows, but when a physician tells him there is no physical basis for his mental and emotional difficulties, what is left but to suppose that he is slowly losing his mind? He may go from one doctor to another—from one kind of tranquilizer to another.

Dr. Stephen Gyland, a Tampa general practitioner who is himself a hypoglycemic, found it terribly difficult to find sound advice. For three years, beginning in 1950, Dr. Gyland went from one specialist to another—fourteen in all—to try to discover why he was chronically anxious, why he had difficulty concentrating. He also suffered physical symptoms: tremors, weakness, dizziness, faintness, and a rapid beating of the heart.

Dr. Gyland was diagnosed as being neurotic by many of these experts. One specialist told him he was definitely *not* neurotic, but that he had a brain tumor. It was not until he happened upon a copy of a 1924 issue of the *Journal of the American Medical Association* that he learned his symptoms were identical to those described by Dr. Seale Harris.

The situation is worse for the layman. Being unable to determine his own problem adequately, he depends on his physician. If the physician does not respect the seriousness of hypoglycemia or is unaware of the disease, his patient's case will become more and more critical.

A college student thought he was losing his mind. Jim Richards began suffering from a variety of symptoms shortly after a bout with the flu. Jim was an engineering major in college when the virus struck in January of 1973.

"For about six months I had been suffering from fatigue," he said. "This was not surprising since I was taking eighteen hours at the university and working after classes and on weekends as a produce manager in a neighborhood grocery. On my doctor's advice, I quit the job and devoted full time to my studies with some left over for relaxation."

Jim thought he had recovered from the viral attack and returned to school. Two days later the fatigue returned. Something was different this time. "I went home from classes to take a nap, a habit that I had never had to develop. Upon awakening I felt dizzy but had an idea that a shower might clear me up. I began to feel faint in the shower and stumbled out in time to call my parents before passing out."

Jim remained in bed for six weeks with a fever that came and went intermittently. He developed a sinus infection that refused to yield to medication. A chronic headache developed during the third week of his bed-bound convalescence, for which the doctor finally prescribed a codeine preparation. Jim developed vertigo.

"At this point I gave up my fight and had my friends check me out of the university for the semester. My emotional stability had collapsed by now and I was deeply depressed, cried easily, and often flew into a rage against the nearest target—the cat or one of my parents. For some unknown reason, I was unable to regain my strength."

Jim visited his family doctor twice a week. Blood and urine tests proved negative, yet Jim still couldn't leave his bed for more than a few minutes without losing what little stored strength he had. "I could still remember my many years of vigorous energy and zest for life and failed to understand why my body had rebelled in this manner, leaving me completely drained and listless."

He had been in bed two months when the sinus infection flared up again. His doctor told him he had a cold, that it was nothing to worry about, and that he should get a job, because his energy would return if he were motivated. "Again I reminded him of the nervousness, anxiety, and fits of rage that still overcame me," said Jim. All Jim needed, his doctor insisted, was a little less worry and a little more interest in life.

Two days after this last visit, Jim tried going out with friends. "I returned early, very ill, in a cold sweat and with nausea. I told my parents that I had lost my mind and that they should put me in a hospital where I wouldn't bother them.

"Terrible fears went through me, especially the fear of insanity. My vision was being affected, things looked distorted. I went to church and realized that shortness of breath prevented me from singing along with the others."

Jim could have gone on like this if he and his parents hadn't begun investigating other physicians. When he came to me I gave him a six-hour glucose-tolerance test, and found him to be severely hypoglycemic.

It took three weeks for the nutritional regimen and medical supervision to take effect.

"My weight has returned to normal and the sinusitis is all but forgotten. The bad days are still there, but they're becoming fewer. I'm back at school; my grades have put me back on the dean's list."

Even if administered, a glucose test may not be interpreted properly. What was immediately required in diagnosing Jim's sickness was a six-hour glucose-tolerance test. But doctors, if they know about the test, often don't like to give it. It requires the loss of a large part of the patient's and the doctor's day. If physicians do give it, sometimes to test for early signs of diabetes, they may only be attentive to the high diabetic levels and not even stop to consider the rapid decline in blood sugar at the end of the test.

The physician administering the test may not even be aware of the seriousness or widespread incidence of hypoglycemia, or know its specific charted signs. If the test proves negative for diabetes, the physician may dismiss the low sugar levels and give the patient a clean bill of health.

A diabetic woman, for instance, had been repeatedly tested by her physician to monitor the progress of her disease. At the third hour her blood sugar was 180 milligrams; she was a mild diabetic. Within another three hours, though, it dropped 140 milligrams to 40 milligrams. Regardless of the abysmal final level, the sheer drop in itself should have been enough to convince any physician that the woman was having hypoglycemic episodes as well as being a diabetic, but her physician considered only the diabetes.

The presence of diabetes can be determined by the analysis of the sugar content in a single drop of a patient's blood. The diagnosis of hypoglycemia would be so much easier if it too were observable in a small sample of blood.

But the doctor who is informed about hypoglycemia isn't totally concerned with the amount of sugar in the blood at any given time. He wants to know how the body reacts to a specific amount of sugar taken orally, that is, he must observe how the body's system handles a sugar solution during several hours of testing.

Thus, low-blood-sugar analysis must consist of a pretest fast of twelve hours, the administration of the sugar-solution test dose, and hourly blood sampling to monitor blood-sugar levels. Urine samples are also checked for sugar during the test to evaluate kidney function as it relates to sugar in the blood.

In a nonhypoglycemic patient, the sugar level will gradually rise and gently fall back to the fasting line.

The normal curve will look like this:

CHART OF NORMAL CURVE

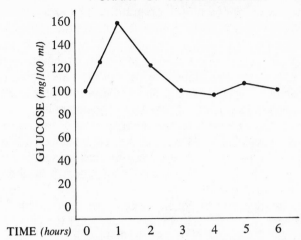

If the patient is hypoglycemic, his curve will not have the gradual rise of the normal chart, but will increase slightly, then drop, often rapidly, until it is well below the fasting level. Also, whatever symptoms the patient has complained of will usually manifest themselves as the test proceeds and his sugar level falls further below normal.

A typical hypoglycemia curve will look something like this:

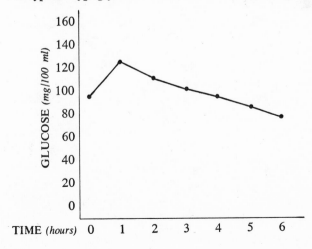

If the test is stopped at the two- or three-hour mark, it may demonstrate the presence of diabetes, but not hypoglycemia. A two- or three-hour glucose-tolerance test usually identifies patients suffering from diabetes, but is too short to record the hypoglycemic episodes that may cause many of the symptoms that are bothering the patient. The diabetic with hypoglycemic episodes will often exhibit a curve that rises above the norm (above 160 milligrams), then sinks rapidly into the hypoglycemic range.

The following graph illustrates how, after the end of two hours, the patient is undeniably diabetic, with an extraordinarily high amount of sugar in his blood. Even his fasting level is high, beginning at 140 milligrams per 100 millimeters of blood, well above the normal 80- to 120-milligram range. If the test had been stopped after two hours, this patient might have been diagnosed solely as a diabetic. But the test was continued, and the patient's blood-sugar level plummeted from 260 milligrams at the two-hour mark to 60 milligrams at the end of five hours, clearly characterizing him as having hypoglycemic episodes as well as diabetes.

CHART OF DIABETIC WITH HYPOGLYCEMIC EPISODES

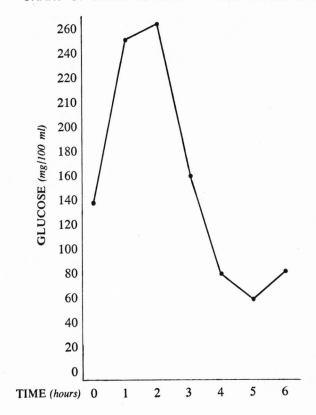

So many of the patients who exhibit this kind of curve are treated only for diabetes, in spite of the fact that they tend not to feel poorly when their sugar levels are high, but suffer allergies, anxieties, fatigue, headaches, or other of the effects of low blood sugar when their levels plunge.

Subclinical hypoglycemia, a product of occupational stress. This form of hypoglycemia produces an entirely different curve, which is basically flat. The blood-sugar content at the beginning of the test is in the normal range, but neither very high nor very low levels occur during the test period. This form of hypoglycemia is particularly difficult to recognize, even with the tolerance test. Many doctors see no significance in the curve, because the levels do not fall below 40 milligrams, which is what many medical articles say is necessary for a medically accepted diagnosis of low blood sugar.

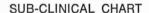

SUB-CLINICAL CHART

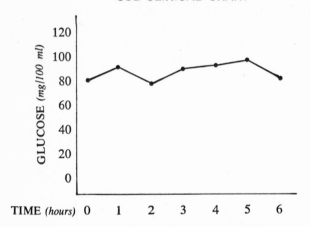

The subclinical form might best be known as the "businessman's disease," because it has often been discovered in young executives who suddenly find their nervous systems at the mercy of arbitrary corporate rise and fall.

American businessmen lead lives of tremendous stress in an environment of constant flux: Ride the wave of advancement or prepare to be fired. To remain in this insecure world can result in a corresponding dislike for the work, and this, in turn, causes a gradual loss of interest and ambition. This lack of ambitious spark in a tense atmosphere can throw the nervous system and the hypothalamus (the master gland of the endocrine system) out of balance. The result is a chronic cycle: The executive's climb to the top frustrated, he worries and becomes restless, his nerves suffer, his blood sugar drops, he becomes fatigued. Coffee, cakes, and martinis worsen the internal energy crisis. Finally, he's at the sub-clinical state; his body, once used to premium fuel, now chugs along on low-octane.

These tired businessmen, Dr. Sydney A. Portis told the American Medical Association, are, "as a rule dependent men whose insecurities and feelings of inferiority are great." He studied fifty of them and found that more than half showed the flat glucose-tolerance curves of the subclinical hypoglycemic. Their complaints usually included a lack of energy, "with boredom and antipathy for their jobs, business superiors and associates."

Subclinical hypoglycemia, of course, is not peculiar to the businessman. It's found in the housewife who is fed up with housework and watching over her mischievous five-year-old. It's found in the inner cities, too, where the constant battle for work and the oppressiveness of poor living conditions create a demoralized outlook among its inhabitants.

Some doctors argue that the blood-sugar level must fall below 40 milligrams by the end of the tolerance test before the patient can actually be considered hypoglycemic. They have been taught that hypoglycemia symptoms will not appear until the sugar level falls below 40 milligrams. Actually, symptoms can appear at far higher levels if the drop occurs rapidly.

Anyone with several of hypoglycemia's symptoms deserves a tolerance test. It is just as important as is an electroencephalograph when a paient suffers from persistent headaches, or a red-blood-cell count when a patient is exhausted. If a five- or six-hour glucose-tolerance test is not proposed, *ask for it.* If your physician doesn't believe in hypoglycemia or does not know how to interpret the graph or treat the disease, search until you find a doctor who *is* capable of diagnosing and treating the disease.[1] If there is even a hint of hypoglycemia, no examination is complete without a prolonged blood-sugar study.

---

[1] Write to the International Academy of Preventive Medicine, 871 Frostwood Drive, Houston, Texas 77024 for a listing of physicians knowledgeable about nutrition and preventive medicine.

Those who do exhibit hypoglycemic symptoms tend to have other medical problems; a total physical examination is necessary to rule out evidence of organic abnormalities. (Too many diagnoses, however, are based on organic changes. If no organic disease is discovered, the doctor concludes there is nothing wrong. Until the doctor can find some definite evidence of organic disease, the patient must wait and suffer.)

An extensive medical history is imperative. Some patients have many of the symptoms of hypoglycemias, yet their tolerance tests prove to be normal. With the aid of their histories, these rare patients—actually suffering metabolic imbalances without the symptoms of low blood sugar—can also be treated with hypoglycemia therapy.

I use computerized questionnaires to focus on the pertinent points of a patient's medical and nutritional history. But even with these questionnaires, it is sometimes difficult to get an accurate history, because so many hypoglycemics are forgetful and easily confused. One patient, I remember, completed her screening interview and had returned for a six-hour glucose test. She entered the office and sat down on a stool that reminded her of a particular stool she had had fifteen years earlier. She then remembered an incident of having blacked out and fallen off that long-ago stool— one of a series of unexplained blackouts she experienced at that time. Her blackouts, one of many signs of the hypoglycemia I found, went unrecorded for fifteen years, and would have gone unrecorded in our history if she had not been reminded by my stool.

Each patient's history should include past and present hereditary, medical, dietary, accident, and surgical information. Some diagnosticians, myself included, sometimes use questionnaires like the one following. This questionnaire lists every possible hypoglycemia symptom, and asks patients to mark any and all symptoms they've experienced. To use it yourself, mark the number "1" next to the symptoms or characteristics you experience mildly, "2" for somewhat strongly, and "3" for severely. When you've finished, add up the figures. Any total above 20 reveals the need of a glucose test.

1. _____ Craving for sweets
2. _____ Craving for candy or coffee in afternoons
3. _____ Craving for alcohol
4. _____ Great consumption of coffee as a pick-me-up
5. _____ Eat often, otherwise get hunger pains or faintness
6. _____ Eat when nervous
7. _____ Hunger between meals
8. _____ "Shaky" when hungry
9. _____ Faintness when meals delayed
10. _____ Fatigue that is relieved by eating
11. _____ Heart palpitations when meals missed or delayed
12. _____ Irritability before meals
13. _____ Sleepy after meals
14. _____ Sleepy during day
15. _____ Feel better after breakfast than before
16. _____ Awaken after few hours sleep—hard to get back to sleep
17. _____ Anxious dreams
18. _____ Afternoon headaches
19. _____ "Butterfly" stomach, cramps
20. _____ Inability to get started in morning before coffee
21. _____ Allergies—tendency to asthma, hay fever, skin rash, etc.
22. _____ Heavy breathing
23. _____ Bleeding gums
24. _____ Spotting or bronzing of skin
25. _____ Blurred vision
26. _____ Inability to make decisions
27. _____ Inability to work under pressure
28. _____ Chronic fatigue
29. _____ Chronic nervous exhaustion
30. _____ Lack of energy
31. _____ Lack of initiative
32. _____ Cry easily for no reason
33. _____ Weakness, dizziness
34. _____ Convulsions
35. _____ Nervous trembling

36. _____ Hand tremors
37. _____ Highly emotional
38. _____ Fearful
39. _____ Hallucinations
40. _____ Dizziness
41. _____ Depression
42. _____ Insomnia
43. _____ Magnify insignificant events
44. _____ Poor memory
45. _____ Worry, feel insecure
46. _____ Moody or melancholy

I will not hesitate to emphasize the flaws in this type of diagnostic method, but it is valuable as a means for patients to recall and focus on any manifestations of their possible metabolic imbalances.

We must remember that hypoglycemia is a great imitator.
It can masquerade as a gastric ulcer or epilepsy, then turn around and imitate schizophrenia.

Thus, the doctor must be extremely wary. If he is not, he will eventually mistreat his patient. Dr. Gyland treated 600 hypoglycemic patients during his career, and found that *320 had been undiagnosed for more than ten years.* Another 133 went untreated for five to ten years. Only one patient in his experience was treated properly a year after becoming ill with hypoglycemia.

In a recent Florida study, 523 patients with hypoglycemia were examined. Five hundred and fourteen were found to have been previously misdiagnosed. Here are the conditions they were diagnosed as having (some patients had several), together with the patient count for each:

DIAGNOSIS	NUMBER
Mentally retarded	15
Slightly nervous, imaginary sickness	76
Neurotic	78
Psychoneurotic	63
Hives	23

Chronic bronchial asthma	75
Skin disease caused by nerves	63
Rheumatoid arthritis	39
Menière's syndrome	5
Parkinson's disease	1
Cerebral arteriosclerosis (*hardening of the arteries in the brain*)	9
Hypertension	24
Menopause	16
Alcoholism	20
Headache	26
Tension headache	21
Postchildbirth shock	19
Diabetes	14
Rapid heartbeat	7

To help in the diagnosis and to track down organic breakdowns, a number of associated blood tests should be used along with the tolerance test. A typical examination could include tests for cholesterol, uric acid, serum calcium, serum chlorides, serum phosphorus, serum sodium, serum glutamic oxalacetic transaminase, lactic dehydrogenase, blood urea nitrogen, creatinine alkaline phosphatase, triglycerides, protein-bound iodine, T_3, T_4, total lipids, and total bilirubin. Hematology studies should include red and white cell count, sedimentation rate, and differential count.

A comprehensive examination should *always* include: a complete urinalysis, an electrocardiogram, a Pap smear test and possibly a cytogram for women, and a prostate-secretion examination for men. Also, both should have a gastric analysis that includes tests for food breakdown.

A patient's hair may be analyzed to determine its cobalt, copper, calcium, iron, lead, lithium, mercury, magnesium, manganese, potassium, and zinc content, and, when necessary, a psychological evaluation should be included.

A comprehensive examination along with a blood-sugar test and a complete history is essential for adequate diagnosis. Once a diagnosis is confirmed, the same programs can become the backbone for the patient's treatment.

The treatment of hypoglycemia is rarely simple. It is a disease that *cannot* be cured, but absolute *control* is possible through a well-rounded medical program designed to reestablish good metabolic and biochemical balance.

The treatment's adequacy rests on a variety of factors: How old is the patient? How long has he or she suffered from hypoglycemia? How badly damaged is the endocrine system? Has there been previous mistreatment and how has it affected the patient?

Effective treatment must take into consideration the specific needs of individual patients, because a chronic, degenerative disease can leave different metabolic, chemical, and hormonal imbalances in each person. While one patient may need drug therapy to reestablish a balance in the nervous system, another may require thyroid for glandular balance. The disease may have struck at the individual's sex-hormone level. Or patients may need treatment to supplement adrenalin production.

The physician must also treat the symptoms of other conditions, if they exist, to relieve the stresses they place on the system. Treatment in these cases may mean chemotherapy, surgery, or psychotherapy. But the basic needs must not be overlooked. An ameliorating drug, such as a tranquilizer, must not be used permanently, but only temporarily while the basic deficiency is corrected.

Just as there is no truly "average" man, there is no "average" hypoglycemic. The infinite genetic pattern present in an individual's chromosomes makes each case different. A subclinical hypoglycemic, for example, cannot be treated as a diabetic with hypoglycemic episodes. He will not improve solely with nutritional augmentation, but must be given psychotherapy to reinstill the zeal and vigor he once felt toward his work. Once the subclinical patient is on a proper diet, however, his psychiatrist can more easily reverse the psychological cycle that make him sick.

Individualized treatment depends on the most accurately focused diagnosis possible. Yet many physicians still treat hypoglycemics with a general approach, in an almost haphazard fashion.

Hypoglycemia is a multifactoral disease, and must be treated as such. Physicians cannot treat low blood sugar as they would a disease that can be cured by eliminating one or two harmful organisms. With hypoglycemia, every factor that either raises or lowers blood sugar must be examined. Doctors who attempt to attribute its cause to a specific factor (the adrenal glands, the insulin level, or the liver) misinterpret the disease. The doctor who treats all of his hypoglycemic patients with adrenal cortex extract (ACE) —a recently devised treatment that seems to be growing in popularity—is also not treating his patients adequately. The adrenal extract may be used only when diagnosis indicates specifically that there is a deficiency in adrenal gland function.

Other misconceptions hinder treatment almost as much as overgeneralizing. Danger exists in the use of large doses of a few vitamins or minerals without balancing them with other nutrients. The concept that diseases have single causes has been a long-standing one in medical philosophy. Unfortunately, some physicians have applied this notion to nutrition and metabolism. They suggest that the intake of a solitary nutrient—or one or two of the most common—will eliminate the problem. This misconception relies on terms such as thiamine deficiency, niacin deficiency, or other statements that suggest that a single nutrient will improve a disease condition.

When thiamine was first presented to the public, it was used widely and in large quantities. Doctors were soon confronted with patients who complained of fatigue and terrible weakness. The use of thiamine without the use of other nutrients produced these harmful effects.

Treatment of blood-sugar levels alone will not control hypoglycemia. The whole patient must be treated. The causes of hypoglycemia rest in the breakdown of nutritionally depleted cells, tissues, and organs. The correction of this metabolic malfunction is essential for recovery and continuing health. When the hypoglycemic's systems are working compatibly again, his condition will be controlled—although his symptoms will quickly return if he wavers from the discipline of the treatment.

The primary objectives in treating hypoglycemia are: alleviation of the vague, distressing symptoms associated with the disease; prevention of the more serious, chronic diseases that hypoglycemia can lead to; and restoration of the carbohydrate-regulating mechanism. "The aim of treatment is to provide the patient with such a clear understanding of his condition that he can recognize any tendency toward a relapse, and thus take steps on his own initiative . . . to avoid severe episodes," notes the Hypoglycemia Foundation, a New York–based nonprofessional group. The patient may help himself by "following the anti-hypoglycemia diet more rigorously, by obtaining more rest, by eliminating the stress factors in his environment, if possible, (or changing his attitude toward them) or by returning to his physician for further treatment and consultation."

Proper treatment should bolster the hypoglycemic's genetic weakness so his cells, tissues, and organs will function as normally as possible. The best method to restore normalcy and to prevent further metabolic deterioration is to increase the amount of proper nutrient intake. This practice usually prevents the genetic deficiency from reappearing.

By making the weakness less evident, the physician will prolong his patient's life. The patient will be less likely to suffer from a chronic, degenerative disease. If a patient is nearsighted, an ophthalmologist will order corrective lenses to strengthen his patient's vision. The lenses will not change the shape of his eyes, but will improve vision by adding support to an area of weakness. Treatment for hypoglycemia works the same way. Nutrient augmentation will support the hypoglycemic's systems enough to compensate for an inherent weakness.

All metabolic processes are controlled by enzymes. Even genetic patterns are perpetuated and expressed through our enzyme systems. These enzyme reactions, however, are dependent upon good nutrition, because the enzymes themselves are made of building blocks the body extracts from food.

Enzyme reactions take place within the cells when the proper nutrients are present. The lack of a single nutrient can disrupt the metabolic chain of enzyme reactions enough to create an imbalance, the first step toward a chronic, degenerative disease. The amino acids, for example, work on a self-limiting basis; the total effect of all the essential amino acids is determined by the amino acid present in the lowest amount. Once that amino acid is exhausted, the chain is broken for all. Other nutrients that the body can neither produce nor store also work on this principle, so it is vitally important regularly to eat foods that contain these materials.

Eating the proper foods may not be enough for the hypo-glycemic. Starved cells, tissues, and organs will not respond to a better diet immediately because, for as yet unexplained reasons, they are unable to absorb or use nutrients as well as their healthy counterparts. Some vitamins and minerals are stored for only a short period, even in healthy tissue. And in deficient tissue they dissipate even more rapidly, especially when the deficiency has caused liver damage or impaired fat digestion.

"Tissues once depleted require much more of the essential factors than it is possible to obtain even in an optimal diet," Canadian physician Morton S. Biskind wrote in *The American Journal of Digestive Diseases.* "It is, nevertheless, important that the diet be as rich in proteins and vitamins as feasible. But the vitamin content of the diet may not be depended on to yield quantities sufficient to heal nutritional lesions [injuries]. Experience indicates that at least ten, twenty, even fifty times the maintenance amounts for persons who have never been deficient are often necessary for therapy, and even after all lesions have healed, the maintenance dosage remains at least five to 10 times the normal intake indefinitely."

In spite of statements such as Dr. Biskind's and other evidence, not enough is being accomplished in nutritional research. Nutrition "plays a role in every medical specialty, [but] financial support from the federal government has been small and largely ineffective and has lagged far behind some of the more dramatic fields," Dr. C. E. Butterworth, chairman of the American Medical Association's Council on Nutrition, told a U.S. Senate committee last year. "Clinical nutrition does not have an identity in the National Institutes of Health, and the chronically underfunded Nutrition Training Grants Program of the N.I.H. has now been discontinued entirely." The lack of such research leaves a gap in both professional and public knowledge and often allows quacks and faddists, who play upon general ignorance, to fill the void.

Why are nutritional supplements necessary? Physicians who have treated a number of hypoglycemics will know from experience that better nutrition alone will not control the disease. Between-meal nutrient supplements must be prescribed, because the patient may have been receiving low amounts of vitamins and minerals, amino acids, and unsaturated fatty acids for years. His depleted tissues must be supplied with large amounts of nutrients so that enough of them will be absorbed until the negative hypoglycemic cycle is reversed.

Part of the hypoglycemic's problem lies in the fact that he handles stress poorly. Researchers have found that these people quickly burn up B-complex vitamins. A high-potency B-complex preparation, therefore, is often used to compensate. One of the better vitamin formulas contains: thiamine (B_1), pantothenic acid, riboflavin (B_2), niacin (B_3), pyridoxine (B_6), B_{12}, C, para-aminobenzoic acid, folic acid and biotin in a base of dessicated liver, brewers' yeast, and kelp. Amounts will vary as patient needs vary.

Minerals should also be added to the hypoglycemic's therapeutic program because they are also necessary for normal metabolic function. A suitable tablet contains: calcium, phosphorus, potassium, dolomite, iron, copper, manganese, magnesium, chromium, and zinc. These should also be taken in a natural base.

A complete, natural, vitamin-mineral tablet should be prescribed with each meal and each snack. Several hundred units of vitamin E should be taken daily, and extra vitamin C to assist the body's immunity mechanism, among its many functions. Extra vitamin A should also be prescribed.

Medication for the digestive system, such as pepsin, betaine, bile salts, bile acids, glutamic acid, and pancreatin—which contains digestive enzymes for breaking down protein, fats, and carbohydrates—may be necessary if the hypoglycemic is not digesting and assimilating his food properly. Other digestive aids may be required. The body can absorb only the smallest and simplest components of food. If gastric secretions, for instance, are not being produced in sufficient quantities to break food down, the hypoglycemic will continue to suffer no matter how much he eats or how much nutritional help is supplied. These medications can be obtained in pharmacies or health-food stores but *should be used only after a physician's recommendations*. It is important that digestive medication be used with between-meal and bedtime snacks, as well as with regular meals. This will assure improved digestion and assimilation.

In many hypoglycemic cases, the liver has been damaged and its sugar-storage capability hindered. Thus choline, methionine, bile salts, bile acids, and inositol may also be necessary as supplements to help regulate liver metabolism. These four materials—lipotrophic agents—support the liver by helping the organ convert fat into glycogen, the sugar compound that is stored in the liver. But lipotrophic agents must be used carefully and with a full complement of other nutrients. Used alone, some investigators think, they can cause cirrhosis.

Again, the hypoglycemic may have been nutrient-deficient for so long that even these oral supplements won't be adequate in restoring the body's absorptive ability. The nutrients may have to be injected. A wilted and dying plant will often not recover if water and fertilizer are placed on the surface. But a hollow rod pushed down into the soil to the roots allows the plant to absorb the nutrients more easily. The body will respond similarly to injections. The absorptive ability will return eventually, and injections can be eliminated.

But no matter what the doctor does, hypoglycemia therapy will fail without the victim's complete cooperation and conscientiousness in following a strict nutritional regimen. The *patient* must fight the craving for sweets. He must pay careful attention to his diet. He must come to grips with stress situations.

The patient and doctor *together* can correct the metabolic imbalance that causes blood-sugar levels to become abnormal. The treatment must be intense, complete, and persistent. It must also be continuous. Hypoglycemia is a chronic disorder capable of reappearing at the slightest lack of cooperation; it demands the greatest degree of nutrition wisdom from the patient who has it and the doctor who treats it.

APPENDICES

The values given in the following tables are of necessity, of course, approximate for average portions. They will be entirely adequate for planning and maintaining good nutrition.

You must know what is in food if you are to become Nutrition-Wise. You need to understand the composition of food to understand calories; and you must learn about the known vitamin and mineral content of foods to practice good nutrition.

Good nutrition is crucial for persons with blood sugar problems. If your cells are deprived of needed nutrients for proper cell metabolism, they are sick cells. If you have sick cells you are a sick person.

Compare these food value tables with the RDA (Recommended Dietary Allowance) keeping in mind the fact that chronically ill persons will require higher amounts than the RDA. The figures are based on a 154 pound male, age 23-50 years of age. Slightly lesser quantities apply to females and children. Older persons also require less total calories.

The menus and recipes based on the role of food components as given in these tables, supply the needed comprehensive information for therapeutic and preventive medicine. The food composition tables offer the information needed to convert regular recipes to Nutrition-Wise ones that are health sustaining. It is easy to change ordinary recipes to ones that contain less fat, carbohydrate and total calories but more nutrients.

Understanding what is in our food today will help you to avoid the acceptance of the fallacy that we are the best fed nation in the world. Your future is in your food. You can make it good or bad.

APPENDIX I
Caloric and Nutritional Values of Common Foods

To understand the value of various foods, you must become familiar with their caloric, vitamin, and mineral content. The following is a listing of common foods together with the calories, carbohydrates, fats, vitamins, and minerals each contains. Use this list as a reference when planning new menus and recipes or converting old favorites (see Appendix III).

GUIDE TO ABBREVIATIONS

CAL.	Calories
CARB.	Carbohydrates (1 gram = 4 cal.)
PROT.	Protein (1 gram = 4 cal.)
SAT.	Saturated fats (1 gram = 9 cal.)
UNSAT.	Unsaturated fats
CA.	Calcium
PHOS.	Phosphorus
SOD.	Sodium
POT.	Potassium
NIA.	Niacin
mg	milligram
IU	International Unit

H	High
M	Medium
L	Low
T	Trace
X	Before fat calories or carbohydrate calories, denotes danger.
TBSP.	tablespoon
TSP.	teaspoon
DIAM.	diameter
QT.	quart
LB.	pound
OZ.	ounce

BERRIES

Berries have a small amount of fat calories and a varying amount of carbohydrate-calorie content. It is fine to use berries without sugar for desserts, appetizers, or snacks. Noncaloric sweetening agents in tablet or liquid form may be used. It is better to use skim milk instead of whole milk or cream with berries, and the sweetening agent may be added to the milk before pouring over the berries.

	MEASURE	CARB.	PROT.	FAT	TOTAL
			Cal.		
Blueberries, fresh	1 Cup	80	5	5	90
Cranberry sauce	1 Cup	x550	—	10	560
Raspberries, black, fresh	1 Cup	80	10	20	110
Raspberries, red, fresh	1 Cup	70	5	5	80
Strawberries, fresh	1 Cup	50	5	5	60

BEVERAGES AND JUICES

Natural juices and beverages are preferred to processed, artificial, or glucose- or sugar-flavored drinks as they contain the important vitamins and minerals and usually have a lower carbohydrate-calorie content. Coffee and tea—no caloric value if taken clear.

	MEASURE	CARB.	PROT.	FAT	TOTAL
			Cal.		
Apple juice	1 Cup	x130	—	—	130
Buttermilk, nonfat	1 Cup	50	35	—	85
Chocolate milk	1 Cup	x110	35	x50	195
Eggnog	6 oz.	70	50	110	230
Ginger ale, dry	1 Cup	x80	—	—	80
Grapefruit juice, unsweetened	1 Cup	x95	5	—	100
Grape juice	1 Cup	x170	5	—	175
Lemon juice	1 tbsp.	5	T	—	5
Milk, evaporated whole	1 Cup	70	180	x100	350
Milk, nonfat dry solids	½ Cup	80	60	—	140
Milk, skim	1 Cup	50	35	—	85
Milk, whole	1 Cup	50	35	x85	170
Orange juice, fresh	1 Cup	105	10	5	120
Orange juice, canned	1 Cup	x140	5	5	150
Orange juice, frozen; diluted with 3 parts water	6 oz.	85	5	—	90
Pineapple juice, canned	1 Cup	x130	5	—	135
Prune juice, canned	1 Cup	x175	5	—	180
Soft drinks, Average	1 Cup	x110	—	—	110
Tomato juice, canned	1 Cup	45	10	5	60
Vegetable juice	1 Cup	85	5	—	90

SAT.	UNSAT.	CA.	PHOS.	IRON	SOD.	POT.	A	B₁	B₂	NIA.	C	D
Fats				*mg.*			*IU*			*mg.*		*IU*
—	—	40	35	2.0	T	200	750	T	T	0.8	50	—
—	—	20	20	1.0	T	40	90	T	T	0.3	5	—
—	—	50	50	1.2	T	300	—	T	T	0.4	30	—
—	—	120	120	2.5	T	350	350	T	T	0.8	75	—
—	—	40	40	1.2	T	300	100	T	T	0.4	100	—

SAT.	UNSAT.	CA.	PHOS.	IRON	SOD.	POT.	A	B₁	B₂	NIA.	C	D
Fats				*mg.*			*IU*			*mg.*		*IU*
—	—	15	20	0.5	5	185	80	T	T	T	5	—
—	—	120	95	0.1	130	140	T	T	0.2	T	T	T
H	L	260	220	0.2	10	80	220	0.1	0.4	0.3	T	5
H	L	250	275	1.5	125	250	850	0.1	0.4	0.2	T	30
—	—	—	—	10.0	10	1	—	—	—	—	—	—
—	—	20	35	0.8	T	375	T	T	T	T	85	—
—	—	15	15	0.5	T	150	—	T	T	T	T	—
—	—	5	5	T	T	—	—	T	T	T	30	—
H	L	500	400	0.4	300	400	550	T	T	T	2	15
—	—	610	425	1.0	35	105	50	0.17	0.8	0.2	5	—
—	—	305	245	T	150	430	T	0.1	0.5	T	5	T
H	L	300	240	2.0	150	420	750	0.1	0.5	T	5	100
—	—	90	40	1.0	10	460	450	T	T	0.5	120	—
—	—	45	50	1.0	1	500	225	T	T	0.5	100	—
—	—	15	30	0.2	T	270	400	0.18	0.02	0.6	90	—
—	—	35	20	0.2	T	300	100	T	T	0.5	20	—
—	—	75	120	0.6	T	500	—	T	T	0.1	5	—
—	—	—	—	—	—	—	—	—	—	—	—	—
—	—	20	40	0.1	600	600	2500	T	T	0.2	40	—
—	—	20	50	0.1	500	500	1700	T	T	T	25	—

BREADSTUFFS

Most of these contain a relatively high carbohydrate content and should be used moderately or restricted, according to your activities and your doctor's nutritional prescription. Beware of spreading these with butter, jellies, preserves, jams, etc. Dietetic jellies and preserves may be used to cut down on carbohydrate calories.

	MEASURE	CARB.	PROT.	FAT	TOTAL
			Cal.		
Biscuit, baking powder	1 small	30	5	10	45
Bread, corn	2"x2"x¾"	50	10	20	80
Bread crumbs	1 Cup	x280	40	30	350
Bread, raisin	1 slice, ½"	50	5	10	65
Bread, rye	1 slice, ½"	50	10	—	60
Bread, white enriched	1 slice, ½"	50	20	5	75
Bread, whole wheat	1 slice, ½"	45	10	5	60
Bun, cinnamon	1 average	105	10	40	155
Bun, hamburger	1 large	170	30	20	220
Crackers, graham	2 medium	40	5	10	55
Crackers, oyster	1 Cup	80	10	25	115
Crackers, saltines	2, 2" square	20	5	5	30
Crackers, soda	2, 2½" square	30	5	10	45
Macaroni, cooked	1 Cup	x170	30	10	210
Macaroni and cheese	1 Cup	x170	70	x220	460
Muffins	1, 2¾" diam.	80	15	35	130
Pancakes	1, 4"	30	5	25	60
Roll	1 average	85	15	10	110
Roll, sweet	1 roll	x120	20	40	180
Spaghetti, cooked	1 Cup	x175	30	10	215
Toast	Same caloric value as bread untoasted				
Toast, cinnamon	1 slice	50	10	50	110
Toast, French	1 slice	110	20	60	190
Toast, melba	1 slice	30	5	5	40
Tortilla	1, 5" diam.	40	5	5	50
Waffle	1, 4½x5⅝"	x110	30	70	210

SAT.	UNSAT.	CA.	PHOS.	IRON	SOD.	POT.	A	B₁	B₂	NIA.	C	D
Fats				*mg.*			*IU*			*mg.*		*IU*
—	—	40	60	1.0	200	40	T	0.1	0.1	0.6	T	—
—	—	30	50	0.5	200	50	50	T	0.1	0.4	T	—
—	—	125	140	3.5	700	150	T	0.2	0.3	3.5	T	—
T	—	35	45	0.6	180	115	T	0.03	0.4	0.3	T	—
T	—	10	60	0.5	—	75	—	0.75	0.03	0.3	—	—
T	—	35	40	1.0	250	40	T	1.2	0.10	1.2	T	—
T	—	50	110	1.2	260	140	T	1.3	0.75	1.4	T	—
T	—	25	40	0.9	300	50	200	0.1	0.1	0.8	—	T
T	—	20	50	1.0	400	60	100	0.2	0.1	1.5	T	—
L	L	10	50	0.3	130	70	—	0.01	0.4	0.3	—	—
—	—	T	6	T	50	—	—	T	T	T	—	—
T	—	T	4	T	20	—	—	T	T	T	—	—
—	—	T	2	T	15	—	—	T	T	T	—	—
—	—	10	50	0.6	—	250	—	T	T	0.4	—	—
M	L	10	150	2.0	1180	130	900	0.2	0.5	2.0	—	T
M	L	50	60	0.6	200	45	50	T	0.1	0.6	—	—
—	—	40	40	0.5	—	—	50	T	T	0.5	—	—
T	—	10	25	0.6	200	30	50	0.1	T	0.8	—	—
T	—	30	50	1.0	—	—	—	0.1	0.1	1.0	—	—
—	—	10	60	1.0	—	—	—	0.15	0.10	1.5	—	—
T	—	35	40	1.0	250	40	T	0.12	0.10	1.2	—	—
T	T	40	50	1.0	250	50	T	0.12	0.10	1.2	—	—
M	L	75	95	1.0	—	—	500	0.1	0.15	0.5	T	10
—	—	30	35	0.5	50	10	—	T	T	T	—	—
—	—	50	40	0.1	—	—	5	0.1	0.1	T	—	—
M	L	200	200	1.8	—	—	360	0.18	0.25	1.3	—	175

CAKES, ICINGS, COOKIES, PIES

All these have too many processed carbohydrates and saturated fat calories and should be avoided.

CAKES

	MEASURE	CARB.	PROT. *Cal.*	FAT	TOTAL
Chocolate layer, 9"	1" wedge	x75	5	x30	110
Coffee cake	small	x200	25	25	250
Cupcake, plain	1, 2¾"	x90	10	x30	130
Doughnut	1	x70	10	x60	140
Fruitcake	1, 2"x2"x½"	70	5	35	110
Plain cake	1, 3"x2"x½"	x125	15	x40	180
Pound cake	1, 2¾" x 3" x ⅝"	60	10	x60	130
Sponge cake, plain, 8"	2" wedge	90	15	20	125

ICINGS

	MEASURE	CARB.	PROT.	FAT	TOTAL
Chocolate	1 tbsp.	x75	5	x30	110
White	1 tbsp.	100	—	—	100

COOKIES

	MEASURE	CARB.	PROT.	FAT	TOTAL
Cookies, plain	1, 3" diam.	x75	5	30	110
Gingersnap	1	10	5	5	20
Macaroon, coconut	1	x20	5	x20	45
Sugar	1	x30	5	20	55

PIES

	MEASURE	CARB.	PROT.	FAT	TOTAL
Apple, 9"	4" wedge	x210	10	x115	335
Blueberry, 9"	4" wedge	x200	10	x80	290
Cherry, 9"	4" wedge	x220	10	x120	350
Chocolate, 9"	4" wedge	x180	40	x240	460
Custard, 9"	4" wedge	x135	30	x100	265
Lemon meringue, 9"	4" wedge	x180	15	x110	305
Mince, 9"	4" wedge	x250	10	85	345
Pumpkin, plain, 9"	4" wedge	x135	20	x115	270

PIE CRUSTS

	MEASURE	CARB.	PROT.	FAT	TOTAL
Single	9" crust	x290	40	x335	665
Double	9" crust	x575	80	x650	1305

SAT.	UNSAT.	CA.	PHOS.	IRON	SOD.	POT.	A	B$_1$	B$_2$	NIA.	C	D
Fats				mg.			*IU*			mg.		*IU*
H	—	20	50	0.5	100	—	160	0.15	0.1	1.5	—	—
M	—	100	150	1.0	300	—	—	0.15	0.1	1.5	—	—
M	—	20	50	0.5	100	—	100	0.15	0.1	1.5	—	—
H	—	70	300	0.7	100	50	150	0.15	0.15	1.2	—	—
L	—	100	125	2.8	100	50	160	0.15	0.15	1.0	—	—
H	—	150	135	0.4	50	50	120	T	T	3.0	—	—
H	—	100	100	0.3	50	50	100	T	T	2.0	—	—
M	—	50	100	0.5	50	50	500	T	1.5	2.0	—	—
H	—	—	—	—	—	—	—	—	—	—	—	—
L	—	—	—	—	—	—	—	—	—	—	—	—
M	—	10	20	T	20	20	10	T	T	T	—	—
L	—	10	20	0.3	100	100	15	T	T	T	—	—
M	—	10	20	0.1	50	50	10	T	T	T	—	—
—	—	10	20	0.1	50	50	10	T	T	T	—	—
H	—	10	25	0.4	300	80	1500	T	T	1.3	—	—
H	—	15	40	0.7	250	80	1500	T	T	2.0	T	—
H	—	15	25	0.3	300	100	450	T	T	0.5	T	—
H	—	70	100	0.7	250	140	200	T	0.1	0.2	T	—
H	—	100	115	0.7	280	140	230	T	0.15	0.3	—	—
H	—	15	50	0.5	280	50	170	T	T	0.2	5	—
H	—	15	40	2.0	400	200	T	T	T	0.4	T	—
H	—	50	80	0.8	200	160	500	T	T	0.1	T	—
H	—	—	—	—	—	—	—	—	—	—	—	—
H	—	—	—	—	—	—	—	—	—	—	—	—

CEREALS

Cereals may be used for breakfast preferably with a tablespoonful of wheat germ and/or ¼ teaspoonful of dry brewers' yeast. Don't forget to add the calories for cream or milk and sugar substitutes on cereals—with 85 for ½ cup of whole milk, 42 for ½ cup of skim milk, and calories for each spoonful of sugar substitute as indicated on the package.

	MEASURE	CARB.	PROT.	FAT	TOTAL
			Cal.		
Bran flakes, all bran	1 Cup	100	30	20	150
Cornflakes	1 Cup	85	10	—	95
Corn grits	1 Cup	110	10	—	120
Cream of Wheat, cooked	1 Cup	120	15	—	135
Oatmeal, cooked	1 Cup	105	20	25	150
Rice, puffed	1 Cup	50	5	—	55
Rice, white, cooked	1 Cup	175	20	—	195
Rice, wild, uncooked	1 Cup	x490	90	10	590
Wheat, puffed	1 Cup	40	5	—	45
Wheat, shredded	1, 4" x 2¼"	90	10	5	105

CHEESE AND EGGS

Cheese and eggs contain protein, minerals, and vitamins but have high fat content. Cottage cheese is the exception and is an excellent choice.

CHEESE

	MEASURE	CARB.	PROT.	FAT	TOTAL
			Cal.		
Blue	1 oz.	—	25	x80	105
Cheddar	1 oz.	—	30	x80	110
Cottage, low-fat, uncreamed	1 Cup	20	175	10	205
Cottage, creamed	1 Cup	40	185	25	250
Cream cheese	1 oz.	—	10	x95	105
Munster	1 oz.	—	30	x85	115
Parmesan	2 tsp.	—	10	10	20
Processed cheese, common * store types*	1 oz.	10	20	x70	100
Swiss (1 sandwich slice)	1 oz.	—	30	x70	100

EGGS

	MEASURE	CARB.	PROT.	FAT	TOTAL
Egg, whole (poached, boiled, * shirred)*	1 medium	—	25	50	75
Egg white	1 medium	—	15	—	15
Egg yolk	1 medium	—	10	50	60

No caloric difference between white and brown eggs.

SAT.	UNSAT.	CA.	PHOS.	IRON	SOD.	POT.	A	B_1	B_2	NIA.	C	D
Fats				*mg.*			*IU*			*mg.*		*IU*
—	—	25	350	3.0	340	300	—	0.2	0.1	5.0	—	400
—	—	5	15	0.5	150	40	—	0.1	0.1	2.0	—	—
—	—	5	25	0.7	5	200	100	0.1	0.1	1.0	—	—
—	—	5	50	0.3	50	T	—	T	T	0.4	—	—
—	—	20	160	1.7	10	130	—	0.2	0.5	0.4	—	—
—	—	—	80	0.3	80	50	—	T	T	0.6	—	—
—	—	45	250	1.6	5	250	—	T	T	1.6	—	—
—	—	20	340	—	5	220	—	0.4	0.6	6.2	—	—
—	—	5	40	0.2	100	30	—	T	T	0.5	—	—
—	—	10	100	0.8	—	—	—	0.6	0.2	1.0	—	—

SAT.	UNSAT.	CA.	PHOS.	IRON	SOD.	POT.	A	B_1	B_2	NIA.	C	D
Fats				*mg.*			*IU*			*mg.*		*IU*
H	—	100	110	0.1	—	—	350	T	0.1	0.1	—	—
H	—	200	140	0.3	190	—	400	T	0.1	T	—	—
L	L	200	400	0.9	600	180	40	0.1	0.6	0.2	—	—
M	L	200	380	0.9	600	170	425	0.1	6.0	0.2	—	—
H	—	20	110	0.1	180	25	440	T	0.1	T	—	—
M	—	180	120	0.1	250	20	350	T	0.1	0.1	—	—
M	—	50	30	T	30	T	50	T	T	T	—	—
—	—	100	150	T	150	—	100	T	T	T	—	—
M	—	250	150	0.3	200	20	400	T	T	0.1	—	—
H	—	50	200	2.7	80	100	1000	0.1	0.3	0.1	—	30
—	—	5	10	—	30	30	—	—	0.15	T	—	—
H	—	20	190	2.7	50	70	100	0.1	1.5	0.1	—	30

DESSERTS

Sugar-containing foods are so high in carbohydrate calories that they seldom should be eaten and if so sparingly. Also, note the amount of fat in some of these foods.

	MEASURE	CARB.	PROT.	FAT	TOTAL
			Cal.		
Butterscotch Pudding	½ Cup	x105	15	60	x180
Custard, Baked	½ Cup	80	30	70	x180
Gelatin, Knox, unflavored	1 envelope	—	30	—	30
Ice Cream	2-oz. scoop	50	10	x70	x130
Ices and sherbets	½ Cup	120	—	—	120
Jell-o desserts	1 average serving	x80	10	—	x90
Malted milk, chocolate	8 oz.	x300	30	50	x380
Malted milk, chocolate, with ice cream	8 oz.	x350	60	100	x510
Pudding, bread, with raisins	¾ Cup	200	30	70	300
Pudding, rice	¾ Cup	210	20	20	x250
Strawberry shortcake	small serving	x215	15	85	x315
Tapioca, cream pudding	½ Cup	80	20	35	135

FATS AND OILS

Avoid fats and oils with high levels of saturated fatty acids. Unsaturated oils are preferred.

	MEASURE	CARB.	PROT.	FAT	TOTAL
			Cal.		
Bacon fat	1 tbsp.	—	—	x100	x100
Butter, salted	1 tbsp.	—	T	x100	x100
Cod liver oil	1 tbsp.	—	—	x125	x125
Corn oil	1 tbsp.	—	—	x125	x125
Cottonseed oil	1 tbsp.	—	—	x125	x125
Cream, light, sweet or sour	1 tbsp.	—	5	x25	x30
Cream, heavy, sweet or sour	1 tbsp.	—	—	x50	x50
Lard	1 tbsp.	—	—	x125	x125
Margarine, Dietetic	1 tbsp.	—	—	50	50
Margarine	1 tbsp.	T	T	x100	x100
Mineral oil	No caloric value				
Olive oil	1 tbsp.	—	—	x125	x125
Peanut oil	1 tbsp.	—	—	x125	x125
Soybean oil	1 tbsp.	—	—	x125	x125
Vegetable shortening	1 tbsp.	—	—	x125	x125

FLOUR

Cornmeal, whole ground	1 Cup	375	45	35	455
Pastry, sifted	1 Cup	x320	30	x10	x360
Rye, sifted	1 Cup	250	30	x10	x290
Soybean, stirred (full fat)	1 Cup	85	105	x135	x325
Whole wheat, sifted	1 Cup	x330	50	x20	x400

SAT.	UNSAT.	CA.	PHOS.	IRON	SOD.	POT.	A	B₁	B₂	NIA.	C	D
Fats				*mg.*			*IU*			*mg.*		*IU*
M	T	160	125	0.8	—	—	200	T	0.2	0.1	—	—
H	M	150	150	0.6	100	200	400	T	0.1	0.1	T	—
—	—	—	—	—	—	—	—	—	—	—	—	—
M	L	100	80	0.1	40	75	330	T	0.1	0.1	5	—
—	—	50	40	—	25	30	—	T	T	—	—	—
—	—	—	—	—	—	—	—	—	—	—	—	—
H	L	350	300	1.0	200	100	700	0.1	0.5	1.0	5	10
H	L	400	375	1.2	250	150	900	0.2	0.5	2.0	5	10
L	—	200	200	1.7	100	200	400	0.1	0.3	0.9	0	5
—	—	200	180	0.6	100	200	200	T	0.2	0.3	T	5
H	L	100	100	2.0	50	100	200	T	0.1	1.0	T	5
H	L	125	125	0.5	200	150	300	T	0.2	0.1	0	0

SAT.	UNSAT.	CA.	PHOS.	IRON	SOD.	POT.	A	B₁	B₂	NIA.	C	D
Fats				*mg.*			*IU*			*mg.*		*IU*
H	—	—	15	0.2	60	5	—	T	T	0.3	—	—
H	—	T	T	—	100	T	400	—	—	T	—	5
L	H	—	—	—	—	—	10,000	—	—	—	—	250
—	H	—	—	—	—	—	—	—	—	—	—	—
—	H	—	—	—	—	—	—	—	—	—	—	—
H	—	15	10	—	5	—	100	T	0.2	T	—	T
H	—	10	10	—	5	—	225	T	0.2	T	—	5
H	—	—	—	—	—	—	—	—	—	—	—	—
L	M	—	—	—	—	—	—	—	—	—	—	—
L	M	—	—	—	—	—	460	—	—	—	—	—
—	—	—	—	—	—	—	T	—	—	—	—	—
L	H	—	—	—	—	—	—	—	—	—	—	—
—	H	—	—	—	—	—	—	—	—	—	—	—
—	H	—	—	—	—	—	—	—	—	—	—	—
H	—	—	—	—	—	—	—	—	—	—	—	—

		CA.	PHOS.	IRON	SOD.	POT.	A	B₁	B₂	NIA.	C	D
—	—	5	225	2.3	T	150	570	3.8	1.0	2.4	—	—
—	—	20	75	0.5	—	100	—	0.3	0.3	0.7	—	—
—	—	50	250	4.5	—	850	—	0.6	0.2	2.7	—	—
—	—	220	1800	8.8	—	1600	100	1.0	0.3	2.9	—	—
—	—	50	450	4.0	5	450	—	0.6	0.2	6.0	—	—

FRUIT

Most canned fruit has sugar added and should be avoided. Use only fresh fruit, canned in natural juices, or dietetic variety. Protein intake can be increased by combining fruit with cottage cheese or unflavored gelatin.

	MEASURE	CARB.	PROT.	FAT	TOTAL
			Cal.		
Apple, raw	1, 2½'' diam.	80	—	—	80
Applesauce	1 Cup	x200	T	5	205
Apricots, raw	3 medium	55	5	T	60
Apricots, canned in syrup	1 Cup	x210	5	5	x220
Apricots, dried cooked, and sweetened	1 Cup	x395	20	5	x420
Banana	1, 6'' x 1½''	x85	5	5	x95
Cantaloupe	½, 5'' diam.	35	5	5	45
Cherries, fresh, raw	1 Cup	65	5	5	75
Cherries, canned	1 Cup	120	10	10	140
Dates, plain	3 medium	75	5	—	80
Figs, fresh	3, 1½'' diam.	x90	5	5	100
Fruit cocktail	1 Cup	x180	5	5	190
Grapefruit	½, 5'' diam.	100	5	5	110
Grapefruit, canned in syrup	1 Cup	x190	5	5	x200
Grapes, raw (slip skin), Concord, etc.	1 Cup	70	10	15	95
Grapes, raw (adherent skin), Muscat, Thompson seedless, Tokay, etc.	1 Cup	105	5	5	115
Honeydew melon	1 wedge, 2'' x 7''	50	5	—	55
Lemon	1 medium, 2¾ x 2''	20	T	5	25
Lime	1 medium, 2'' diam.	25	—	—	25
Mango, raw	1 medium	90	5	5	100
Nectarine	1 medium	80	5	—	85
Orange	1 medium, 3''	70	5	5	80
Papaya, raw	½ medium	75	5	—	80
Peach, raw	1 medium	80	5	—	85
Peaches, canned	1 Cup	x185	5	5	195
Pear, fresh	1 medium	120	5	5	130
Pears, canned in syrup	2 medium	x190	—·	5	195
Pineapple, raw	1 slice, 3½'' x 3¾''	45	—	5	50
Pineapple, canned in syrup	1 slice (large)	x100	—	—	x100
Plum, raw	1, 2'' diam.	30	—	—	30
Plums, canned in syrup	1 Cup	x190	5	—	195
Prunes, dried	6 medium	170	—	—	170
Raisins, dried	1 Cup	x450	10	5	465
Tangerine	1, 2½'' diam.	90	10	5	105
Watermelon	½'' slice, 6'' x 1½''	145	5	10	160

SAT.	UNSAT.	CA.	PHOS.	IRON	SOD.	POT.	A	B₁	B₂	NIA.	C	D
	Fats			*mg.*			*IU*			*mg.*		*IU*
—	—	5	10	0.3	T	75	100	T	T	0.2	15	—
—	—	10	20	1.0	T	100	80	T	T	0.2	T	—
—	—	15	25	0.5	—	450	2800	T	T	0.8	10	—
—	—	30	35	8.0	—	600	4500	T	T	0.9	10	—
—	—	200	200	9.0	30	1500	6000	T	T	2.5	25	—
—	—	10	30	6.0	—	400	450	T	T	0.7	10	—
—	—	15	15	0.4	10	225	3500	T	T	0.5	30	—
—	—	20	20	1.0	—	250	600	T	T	0.4	10	—
—	—	20	20	1.0	10	600	700	T	T	0.5	10	—
—	—	20	20	0.6	T	25	20	T	T	0.7	—	—
—	—	55	30	0.6	T	200	80	T	T	0.5	0.5	—
—	—	20	25	0.8	T	200	180	T	T	0.8	5.0	—
—	—	40	20	0.4	T	400	—	T	T	0.4	75	—
—	—	45	45	0.6	—	400	10	T	T	0.4	60	—
—	—	35	40	1.0	10	160	160	T	0.1	0.4	10	—
—	—	50	60	1.5	15	400	200	T	0.1	0.5	15	—
—	—	25	25	4.0	—	—	40	T	T	0.2	50	—
—	—	40	20	0.6	T	130	—	T	T	0.1	50	—
—	—	40	20	0.6	—	100	—	T	T	0.19	25	—
—	—	10	15	0.2	—	—	6300	T	T	0.9	40	—
—	—	—	—	0.5	—	300	1500	T	T	T	25	—
—	—	50	35	0.6	T	300	300	T	T	0.2	75	—
—	—	40	30	0.5	10	475	3500	T	T	0.6	110	—
—	—	10	25	0.6	T	150	900	T	T	0.9	10	—
—	—	10	35	0.8	T	300	1100	T	T	6.0	110	—
—	—	15	30	0.5	T	180	30	T	T	0.2	10	—
—	—	10	40	0.2	10	60	T	0.1	0.1	0.2	0	—
—	—	15	10	0.3	T	200	110	0.1	T	0.2	20	—
—	—	30	10	0.7	T	150	100	0.1	T	0.2	100	—
—	—	10	20	0.3	T	100	200	T	T	0.3	5	—
—	—	10	10	1.0	20	110	1000	T	T	0.4	T	—
—	—	T	T	2.0	300	5	473	0.08	0.02	1.5	T	—
—	—	T	5	0.3	1020	40	100	0.16	0.04	0.2	T	—
—	—	35	25	0.4	T	100	400	0.1	T	0.2	30	—
—	—	40	70	1.2	T	600	5000	0.3	0.3	1.8	5	—

MEATS AND FOWL

Caloric values listed are approximate and for meats with excess fat trimmed before cooking. Frying or panbroiling is not permissible because the fat cannot drain out of the cooked meat. So, broil, bake, roast, boil, or barbecue your meats.

	MEASURE	CARB.	PROT.	FAT	TOTAL
				Cal.	
Bacon, broiled crisp	2 slices	—	15	80	95
Bacon, Canadian	4 oz.	—	100	x150	250
Beef, corned, lean	3 oz.	—	90	60	150
Beef, dried or chipped	3 oz.	—	115	50	165
Beef, ground, lean	3 oz.	—	90	100	190
Beef, roast, rib	3 oz.	—	80	185	265
Beef, sirloin	3 oz.	—	80	170	250
Beef, tenderloin	3 oz.	—	130	95	225
Bologna, all beef	1 slice 4" x ½" x ⅛"	5	40	50	95
Bologna, regular	1 slice 1" x 1½"	30	120	x300	450
Chicken, roasted	4 oz.	—	90	130	220
Chicken livers	3 oz.	10	75	30	115
Duck, lean roasted portion	4 oz.	—	125	40	165
Frankfurter, all beef	1 average	5	60	45	110
Frankfurter, regular	1 average	5	30	x90	125
Ham, baked (lean)	3 oz.	—	110	30	140
Ham, boiled	3 oz.	—	75	175	250
Ham, canned, spiced	3 oz.	5	50	x180	235
Ham, deviled	1 tbsp.	—	15	60	75
Hash, corned beef	3 oz.	25	45	45	115
Lamb chops, rib (medium fat)	3 oz.	—	80	x270	350
Lamb, leg of, roasted	3 oz.	—	80	140	220
Lamb, shoulder, roasted	3 oz.	—	70	x215	285
Liver, beef or calf	3 oz.	35	80	55	170
Liver, chicken	3 oz.	10	75	30	115
Liverwurst	2 oz.	5	40	x105	150
Meat loaf, beef & pork	1 average slice, 3 oz.	45	50	x175	270
Pork chop, broiled, lean	1 average, 3 oz.	—	80	x205	285
Pork, ribs, roasted	3 ribs, 2 oz.	—	35	90	125
Pork, roast, loin	3 oz.	—	80	x200	280
Pork sausage, link or bulk	4 oz.	—	50	x450	500
Turkey, roasted (light or dark meat)	3 oz.	—	150	40	190
Veal, cutlet, broiled	3 oz.	—	95	80	175
Veal, leg, roast	3 oz.	—	110	100	210
Veal, shoulder, roast	3 oz.	—	95	90	185

SAT.	UNSAT.	CA.	PHOS.	IRON	SOD.	POT.	A	B_1	B_2	NIA.	C	D
Fats				mg.			IU			mg.		IU
L	M	5	40	0.5	400	50	—	0.1	T	0.5	—	—
L	M	10	180	3.0	2000	350	—	0.8	0.25	5.0	—	—
H	H	20	100	4.3	1300	50	—	T	T	3.5	—	—
L	L	15	300	1.5	3000	150	—	T	0.2	3.0	—	—
L	L	10	160	3.0	120	350	20	T	T	5.5	—	—
H	L	10	175	3.0	100	350	—	T	0.1	4.5	—	—
M	M	10	150	2.5	60	320	30	T	T	4.0	—	—
M	M	10	150	3.0	40	350	20	T	0.3	2.5	—	—
H	L	10	100	2.5	800	200	—	T	T	3.0	—	—
H	L	10	100	2.2	1100	220	—	T	T	2.5	—	—
L	H	20	200	1.7	100	350	—	0.1	0.2	10.0	—	—
H	L	15	240	7.5	75	300	32,000	0.2	2.5	11.8	20	50
M	H	20	220	8.0	100	325	—	0.1	2.5	7.0	—	—
M	L	5	25	0.5	400	100	—	0.2	0.2	2.5	—	—
H	L	5	25	0.5	500	100	—	0.1	0.1	1.2	—	—
H	T	10	200	2.0	900	400	—	0.7	0.2	4.0	—	—
H	L	5	250	2.3	50	400	—	0.5	0.1	4.0	—	—
H	L	5	250	2.3	750	300	—	0.3	0.1	3.0	—	—
H	L	T	20	0.5	—	—	—	—	—	5.0	—	—
M	L	20	100	4.3	—	—	—	—	0.2	1.5	—	—
H	L	10	80	0.3	80	500	—	0.2	0.3	8.0	—	—
H	L	25	200	3.0	80	500	—	0.2	0.3	7.0	—	—
H	L	10	200	3.0	80	500	—	0.2	0.3	7.0	—	—
H	L	10	350	6.6	80	325	45,000	0.2	3.3	13.7	30	50
H	L	15	240	7.5	75	300	32,000	0.2	2.5	11.8	20	50
H	L	10	240	5.4	—	—	5100	0.1	1.0	4.6	—	15
H	L	10	175	1.8	—	—	—	0.1	0.2	2.5	—	—
H	L	10	250	5.0	60	500	—	1.0	1.5	5.0	—	—
H	L	5	100	1.0	25	225	—	0.2	0.1	1.0	—	—
H	L	5	300	4.5	50	500	—	1.2	0.3	4.5	—	—
H	L	10	150	2.0	800	200	—	0.6	0.2	3.0	—	—
L	H	30	400	5.0	—	—	10	T	0.1	9.0	—	—
L	M	10	200	3.5	50	400	—	—	—	—	—	—
L	M	10	250	4.0	75	500	—	0.1	0.2	8.0	—	—
L	M	10	250	4.0	50	500	—	0.1	0.3	6.0	—	—

MISCELLANEOUS

These foods contain a varying amount of calories. Some are flavoring agents. Many of these foods can be used to increase the appetite appeal or improve the taste of many dishes.

	MEASURE	CARB.	PROT.	FAT	TOTAL
			Cal.		
Bouillon cube	1 cube	—	5	—	5
Catsup	1 tbsp.	20	—	—	20
Caviar, granular	2 tbsp.	—	20	25	45
Chili sauce	1 tbsp.	15	—	—	15
Chocolate, baking, unsweetened	1 oz.	35	5	x135	175
Chocolate, sweet	1 oz.	70	—	75	145
Cornstarch	1 tbsp.	30	—	—	30
Croutons	5 1-oz. cubes	50	10	55	115
Dressing, poultry, bread	⅓ Cup	90	15	60	165
French dressing	1 tbsp.	10	—	50	60
Gravy	1 tbsp.	—	—	50	50
Gum, chewing	1 stick	15	—	—	15
Hard sauce	1 tbsp.	50	—	—	50
Hollandaise sauce	2 tbsp.	—	—	155	155
Horseradish	2 tsp.	5	—	—	5
Lecithin granules	2 tbsp.	—	—	100	100
Mayonnaise	1 tbsp.	—	—	90	90
Mustard, prepared	1 tsp.	—	—	—	—
Olives, green	10 large	10	5	60	75
Olives, black	10 large	5	5	105	115
Peanut butter	1 tbsp.	15	15	70	100
Pickles, dill	1 large	10	5	5	20
Pickles, sweet	2, 2" x ⅝"	20	—	—	20
Pimentos	1 tbsp.	5	—	—	5
Popcorn, popped	1 Cup	40	5	5	50
Potato chips	7 large, 3" diam.	40	5	65	110
Potato salad	½ Cup	65	10	145	220
Pretzels	5 small sticks	15	—	—	15
Vinegar	1 tbsp.	5	—	—	5
Wheat germ	1 tbsp.	15	10	5	30
White sauce	1 Cup	95	40	x300	435
Yeast, compressed, bakers'	1 cake	15	10	—	25
Yeast, dried, brewers'	1 tbsp.	10	20	—	30
Yogurt, plain	½ Cup	20	15	20	55

SAT.	UNSAT.	CA.	PHOS.	IRON	SOD.	POT.	A	B₁	B₂	NIA.	C	D
Fats				mg.			IU			mg.		IU
—	—	—	—	0.1	100	10	—	—	—	—	—	—
H	L	5	5	0.1	200	100	300	T	T	T	—	—
M	L	80	100	2.0	100	25	—	—	—	—	—	—
—	—	—	5	0.1	—	—	300	T	T	T	—	—
H	L	25	125	3.0	—	300	20	T	T	0.1	—	—
H	L	20	80	1.8	10	65	10	T	T	0.2	—	—
—	—	—	—	—	T	T	—	—	—	—	—	—
M	L	—	—	—	—	—	—	—	—	—	—	—
—	—	40	50	0.3	200	50	T	T	T	0.1	—	—
L	H	T	T	T	—	—	—	—	—	—	—	—
H	—	10	5	—	50	20	—	—	—	—	—	—
M	T	—	—	—	T	T	—	—	—	T	—	—
H	T	25	75	0.9	—	—	900	T	T	T	—	—
—	H	T	500	T	T	T	—	—	—	—	—	—
M	M	—	10	0.1	—	—	35	T	T	T	—	—
L	H	50	10	1.0	900	30	150	T	T	T	—	—
L	H	50	10	1.0	900	30	100	T	T	T	—	—
H	—	15	80	0.4	25	150	—	T	T	3.2	—	—
—	—	50	40	1.2	1500	300	300	T	T	T	—	—
—	—	5	5	0.1	—	—	10	T	T	T	—	—
—	—	5	5	0.5	—	—	800	T	T	T	—	—
—	—	5	40	0.4	200	35	—	T	T	T	—	—
—	—	5	15	0.2	35	80	5	T	T	0.3	—	—
T	M	20	50	0.8	—	—	250	T	T	0.8	15	—
—	—	10	110	0.8	—	—	40	0.2	0.1	0.5	—	10
H	L	300	250	0.6	—	—	1300	0.1	0.4	0.7	T	—
—	—	5	50	0.3	—	40	—	0.1	0.2	2.8	—	—
—	—	20	150	1.9	15	150	—	1.6	0.6	3.3	—	—
L	L	175	125	T	65	150	75	0.1	0.2	0.1	—	—

NUTS

All values are for shelled nuts. Fat content is high.

	MEASURE	CARB.	PROT.	FAT	TOTAL
			Cal.		
Almonds	10	10	10	x70	90
Brazil	4	20	20	x90	130
Cashews, dry-roasted	1 oz.	25	20	50	95
Chestnuts	5	55	5	5	65
Coconut, shredded	1 Cup	130	10	x220	360
Filberts, Hazel	10	10	5	x75	90
Peanuts, dry-roasted	1 oz.	25	30	45	100
Pecans, chopped	1 tbsp.	5	5	50	60
Soybeans, dry roasted	1 oz.	30	55	60	145
Walnuts, chopped	1 tbsp.	5	5	45	55

SAT.	UNSAT.	CA.	PHOS.	IRON	SOD.	POT.	A	B₁	B₂	NIA.	C	D
Fats				*mg.*			*IU*			*mg.*		*IU*
T	H	30	70	0.6	T	100	—	T	0.1	0.4	—	—
H	L	30	100	0.5	T	300	—	0.1	—	—	—	—
T	L	15	107	1.0	25	140	—	0.17	0.4	0.7	—	—
—	H	5	15	0.3	T	60	—	T	T	0.1	—	—
H	T	25	120	0.2	10	500	—	T	T	0.4	—	—
M	M	40	50	0.5	T	70	15	T	T	1.1	—	—
M	T	25	135	0.7	T	230	—	0.10	0.4	5.7	—	—
—	—	10	50	0.4	T	60	10	0.1	T	0.1	T	—
T	T	50	140	1.0	125	275	T	0.33	0.1	0.7	—	—
—	H	5	30	0.2	T	35	T	T	T	0.1	T	—

SEAFOOD

Seafood and fish are excellent choices; they are usually high in protein and low in fat, unless fried. Shellfish is especially high in minerals.

	MEASURE	CARB.	PROT.	FAT	TOTAL
			Cal.		
Abalone	1, 6″ fillet, 3 oz.	—	55	20	75
Bass, black, baked	4 oz.	—	130	100	230
Bluefish, broiled	4 oz.	—	135	45	180
Carp, broiled	4 oz.	—	100	30	130
Clams, shelled	3 oz.	5	30	10	45
Codfish cakes, baked	2 small, 3 oz.	20	15	60	95
Codfish steak, steamed	4 oz.	—	95	5	100
Crab, canned or cooked	3 oz.	5	60	20	85
Haddock, steamed	1 fillet, 3 oz.	—	95	5	100
Halibut, broiled	1 fillet, 3 oz.	—	130	90	220
Herring, pickled	1 fillet, 3 oz.	—	80	x135	215
Lobster, canned meat	3 oz.	—	65	10	75
Lobster, broiled	4 oz.	—	80	10	90
Mackerel, canned	3 oz.	—	70	75	145
Mackerel, fresh, broiled	3 oz.	15	80	65	160
Oysters, shelled	1 Cup, 6 oz.	55	95	45	195
Perch, fried	1 fillet	—	60	50	110
Salmon, canned, red	3 oz.	—	70	75	145
Salmon, fresh, broiled	3 oz.	—	90	10	100
Sardines, canned in oil	3 oz.	5	70	x200	275
Sardines, canned in tomato sauce	3 oz.	5	60	115	180
Scallops	3 oz.	10	80	5	95
Shrimp, fresh, boiled	3 oz.	—	65	5	70
Trout, steamed or broiled	1, 7 oz.	10	170	45	225
Tuna, canned in oil	3 oz.	—	80	160	240
Tuna, canned, water-pack	3 oz.	—	80	50	130
White bass, steamed	4 oz.	—	100	15	115
Whitefish, broiled	3 oz.	—	80	10	90

SAT.	UNSAT.	CA.	PHOS.	IRON	SOD.	POT.	A	B₁	B₂	NIA.	C	D
Fats				mg.			IU			mg.		IU
L	H	35	200	2.5	—	—	—	T	T	—	—	—
T	H	100	250	1.5	50	250	100	0.1	0.2	4.0	—	5
T	H	30	300	1.0	75	—	50	0.1	0.1	1.0	—	50
L	H	50	250	1.0	50	250	175	T	T	0.5	—	10
L	H	100	150	7.0	200	250	100	0.1	0.2	1.5	—	10
L	H	50	200	0.6	200	200	50	T	0.1	2.0	—	5
L	H	30	200	0.5	300	300	20	T	0.1	2.5	—	5
L	H	50	180	1.0	800	100	20	T	T	2.0	—	5
L	H	20	150	0.6	—	—	100	T	T	2.0	—	—
L	H	15	250	0.8	50	500	100	0.1	0.1	10.0	—	—
L	H	10	—	1.0	—	—	50	T	T	1.0	—	—
L	M	50	150	0.7	—	—	500	T	T	20.0	—	—
L	H	100	200	0.7	200	200	1000	0.1	T	2.5	—	—
L	H	200	250	2.0	—	—	500	T	T	5.0	—	—
L	H	100	250	—	—	—	—	—	—	—	—	—
M	M	200	350	13.0	75	100	300	0.1	0.2	1.2	—	—
H	—	10	100	0.7	—	—	—	T	T	2.5	—	—
T	H	175	300	1.0	75	300	300	T	0.15	8.5	—	10
T	H	150	300	1.2	100	400	200	T	T	8.0	—	10
L	H	300	400	3.0	400	450	200	T	0.1	4.0	—	100
L	H	400	200	4.5	400	300	50	T	0.2	5.5	—	50
L	H	100	300	3.0	250	475	50	—	T	1.3	—	10
L	H	100	250	1.5	150	150	20	—	T	2.0	—	10
L	H	25	250	1.2	—	—	20	T	T	3.5	—	10
L	H	10	300	1.2	—	—	20	T	0.1	12.0	—	10
L	H	10	350	1.4	—	—	20	T	0.1	12.0	—	10
T	H	100	250	1.5	50	250	75	0.1	0.2	4.0	—	5
L	H	75	250	1.3	50	300	20	0.1	0.1	4.0	—	10

SOUPS

Avoid creamed soups; use clear soups. Bouillon and consomme are excellent sources of protein. They are high in satiety value (hunger-satisfying) and contain very little fat. These calculations are based on adding whole milk to commercial canned creamed soups.

	MEASURE	CARB.	PROT.	FAT	TOTAL
			Cal.		
Bean, Yankee	1 Cup	120	35	45	200
Beef broth	1 Cup	45	25	30	100
Bouillon, canned	1 Cup	5	25	—	30
Chicken broth	1 Cup	40	15	25	80
Clam chowder	1 Cup	50	20	20	90
Consomme	1 Cup	—	35	—	35
Mushroom, cream of	1 Cup	50	30	120	200
Onion	1 Cup	30	20	55	105
Oyster, with milk	1 Cup	40	40	90	170
Potato, cream of	1 Cup	45	15	45	105
Split pea	1 Cup	100	25	20	145
Tomato, cream of	1 Cup	45	15	60	120
Vegetable (no meat or fat)	1 Cup	60	15	15	90

SWEETS

Sugar-containing foods are so high in carbohydrate-calorie count that they should seldom be eaten and then very sparingly. Also, note the amount of fat in some of these foods.

	MEASURE	CARB.	PROT.	FAT	TOTAL
			Cal.		
Caramels	1 oz.	90	5	30	x125
Carob powder	1 oz.	10	5	95	110
Chocolate bar, plain	2 squares	80	—	20	x100
Chocolate fudge	1 oz.	90	—	30	x120
Chocolate syrup	1 oz.	60	5	5	x70
Cocoa, dry	1 tbsp.	10	—	10	20
Corn syrup	1 tbsp.	60	—	—	x60
Gumdrop	1, 1½'' diam.	30	5	—	35
Hard candy	average piece	30	—	—	30
Honey	1 tbsp.	65	—	—	65
Jam and jelly	1 tbsp.	60	—	—	60
Jelly beans	4	30	—	—	30
Maple sugar	1 tbsp.	50	—	—	x50
Marshmallow	1 oz.	90	—	—	90
Molasses	1 tbsp.	50	—	—	50
Peanut brittle	1 oz.	80	10	x40	x130
Powdered sugar	1 tbsp.	30	—	—	30
Sugar, brown, firm	1 tbsp.	50	—	—	50

SAT.	UNSAT.	CA.	PHOS.	IRON	SOD.	POT.	A	B₁	B₂	NIA.	C	D
	Fats			*mg.*			*IU*			*mg.*		*IU*
—	—	50	100	2.0	80	300	500	0.1	—	—	—	—
—	—	—	25	0.2	750	100	—	—	—	0.2	—	—
—	—	—	25	0.2	750	100	—	—	—	0.2	—	—
—	—	—	—	—	500	—	—	—	—	—	—	—
—	—	25	50	0.9	700	700	700	—	—	0.9	—	—
—	—	—	25	0.2	700	100	—	—	—	0.2	—	—
M	L	150	100	0.5	800	100	100	—	0.1	0.3	—	—
—	—	25	25	0.4	850	75	—	—	—	—	—	—
H	L	250	200	1.0	700	100	200	0.1	0.2	0.4	—	—
—	—	50	50	0.7	900	—	300	—	—	0.4	—	—
—	—	10	50	0.6	300	100	200	0.1	—	0.6	—	—
—	—	100	75	0.5	750	100	100	—	—	0.5	—	—
—	—	50	30	0.6	500	100	2000	0.1	0.2	0.9	—	—

SAT.	UNSAT.	CA.	PHOS.	IRON	SOD.	POT.	A	B₁	B₂	NIA.	C	D
	Fats			*mg.*			*IU*			*mg.*		*IU*
M	L	35	40	0.7	40	50	10	—	—	—	—	—
—	—	70	40	1.6	—	315	15	T	T	0.8	—	—
H	L	50	60	0.7	30	100	40	—	—	—	—	—
H	L	30	40	0.4	70	50	—	—	—	—	—	—
H	L	5	25	0.6	15	50	—	—	—	—	—	—
M	L	10	50	0.5	100	—	—	T	T	0.2	—	—
—	—	10	T	0.6	—	—	—	—	—	T	—	—
—	—	—	—	—	—	—	—	—	—	—	—	—
—	—	—	—	—	—	—	—	—	—	—	—	—
—	—	T	T	0.2	T	T	5	T	T	0.1	5	—
—	—	T	T	T	T	T	T	T	T	T	T	—
—	—	—	—	—	—	—	—	—	—	—	—	—
—	—	—	—	—	—	—	—	—	—	—	—	—
—	—	T	T	T	T	T	—	—	—	—	—	—
—	—	100	20	2.5	—	—	—	0.1	0.2	0.5	—	—
—	—	10	30	0.5	—	—	5	0.1	T	1.0	—	—
—	—	—	—	—	—	—	—	—	—	—	—	—
—	—	20	10	0.2	10	50	—	—	—	—	—	—

VEGETABLES

Vegetables are good sources of vitamins, minerals, and cellulose. Cellulose supplies roughage for the intestinal tract and tends to provide bulk, which satisfies hunger. The proteins of vegetables are not considered primary or complete proteins except those of soybeans.

	MEASURE	CARB.	PROT.	FAT	TOTAL
			Cal.		
Artichoke	1 medium	10	5	—	15
Asparagus, canned	6 tips	15	10	5	30
Asparagus, fresh, cooked	6 tips	5	5	5	15
Avocado	½ med., 3½'' x 3½''	20	5	x270	295
Beans, baked with pork (sweet)	1 Cup	185	60	50	295
Beans, wax, canned or cooked	1 Cup	20	5	—	25
Beans, kidney, canned or cooked	1 Cup	160	60	10	230
Beans, lima, green, cooked	1 Cup	130	40	5	175
Beans, string, green, canned or cooked	1 Cup	25	5	—	30
Beets, not buttered	1 Cup	60	5	—	65
Beet greens, cooked	1 Cup	30	10	5	45
Broccoli	1 Cup	35	10	5	50
Brussels sprouts	1 Cup	45	15	5	65
Cabbage, raw	1 Cup	20	5	—	25
Carrots, raw	1 Cup	40	5	5	50
Cauliflower, raw	1 Cup	20	10	—	30
Celery, raw	1 large stalk	15	5	—	20
Chives	1 Cup	25	15	5	45
Corn, white or yellow, fresh	1, 5'' ear	80	10	5	95
Corn, canned	1 Cup	135	25	10	170
Cucumbers, raw	1, 7½'' x 2''	20	5	—	25
Eggplant, steamed	1 Cup	20	5	—	25
Endive, raw	2 oz.	10	5	—	15
Hominy	1 Cup	105	10	—	115
Lettuce, iceberg	1-lb. head	55	20	5	80
Lettuce, romaine	5 large leaves	5	5	—	10
Mushrooms, cooked or canned	1 Cup	35	10	5	50
Okra, cooked	8 pods	25	5	—	30
Onions, raw, chopped	1 tbsp.	5	—	—	5
Onions, cooked	1 Cup	75	10	5	90
Parsley, raw, chopped	1 tbsp.	—	—	—	—
Parsnips, cooked	1 Cup	85	5	5	95
Peas, black-eyed, cooked	1 Cup	100	45	10	155
Peas, canned	1 Cup	110	30	10	150

SAT.	UNSAT.	CA.	PHOS.	IRON	SOD.	POT.	A	B$_1$	B$_2$	NIA.	C	D
Fats				mg.			IU			mg.		IU
—	—	40	50	1.0	40	400	50	0.1	0.1	0.1	—	—
—	—	20	50	2.0	200	250	800	0.1	0.1	1.0	—	—
—	—	20	50	1.0	10	150	600	0.1	0.2	1.2	—	—
T	H	10	40	5.0	10	1500	7500	T	0.1	3.0	10	—
L	—	70	140	2.5	500	200	150	T	T	0.7	—	—
—	—	35	25	0.7	10	150	650	T	T	0.5	—	—
—	—	40	125	2.0	10	900	—	0.1	0.1	0.2	—	—
—	—	50	125	3.0	—	400	250	T	T	2.0	—	—
—	—	35	25	2.2	—	150	750	T	T	0.5	—	—
—	—	25	45	1.0	60	300	30	T	T	0.5	—	—
—	—	200	100	6.5	250	550	6000	T	0.1	0.3	30	—
—	—	200	100	2.1	15	400	5000	T	0.2	0.5	10	—
—	—	50	90	1.7	15	400	500	T	0.1	0.6	60	—
—	—	50	30	T	10	450	80	T	T	0.2	—	—
—	—	40	30	1.0	400	30	13,000	T	T	0.7	10	—
—	—	30	100	1.2	10	200	80	T	T	0.6	30	—
·	—	20	20	0.2	30	100	0.2	T	T	0.2	5	—
—	—	140	80	3.4	—	500	5850	T	T	0.2	100	—
—	—	5	120	0.5	T	300	300	T	T	1.1	10	—
—	—	10	100	1.3	500	400	500	T	T	2.4	15	—
—	—	10	20	0.3	10	200	—	T	T	0.1	5	—
—	—	15	60	1.0	—	400	10	T	T	0.9	10	—
—	—	45	30	1.0	10	250	1500	T	T	0.1	5	—
—	—	—	10	0.5	—	10	60	T	T	0.4	—	—
—	—	140	150	1.6	75	800	5000	0.3	0.5	1.0	50	—
—	—	40	15	0.8	10	75	900	T	T	0.1	10	—
—	—	15	150	1.5	600	300	—	T	0.6	6.0	5	—
—	—	70	50	0.6	—	350	750	T	T	0.7	20	—
—	—	5	5	—	—	—	5	T	T	T	T	—
—	—	60	70	0.5	15	300	—	—	—	0.4	20	—
—	—	20	10	0.4	—	50	300	T	T	0.1	10	—
—	—	90	100	1.1	10	575	—	T	0.2	0.3	20	—
—	—	20	100	2.2	—	200	650	0.2	T	1.5	20	—
—	—	20	120	1.8	—	200	900	0.3	T	1.5	15	—

VEGETABLES (continued)	MEASURE	CARB.	PROT.	FAT	TOTAL
				Cal.	
Peas, green, cooked	1 Cup	75	30	5	110
Pepper, green, raw	1 large	15	5	—	20
Potato, baked in jacket	1 medium	90	10	—	100
Potato, boiled	1 medium	95	10	—	105
Potato chips	10 medium	40	5	x65	110
Potato, French fried	8 medium	85	10	70	165
Potato, hash-browned	1 Cup	240	25	x205	470
Potato, mashed, milk added	1 Cup	135	15	15	165
Potato, sweet, boiled	1 medium	160	10	10	180
Potato, sweet, candied	1 medium	250	10	55	315
Pumpkin, canned	1 Cup	70	10	5	85
Radishes	4 small	5	—	—	—
Rhubarb, cooked, sweetened	1 Cup	390	5	5	400
Sauerkraut, canned	1 Cup	30	10	5	45
Soybeans, cooked	1 Cup	90	80	90	260
Soybeans, sprouts	1 Cup	25	25	15	65
Spinach, cooked, fresh or canned	1 Cup	25	20	10	55
Squash, summer variety, soft shell	1 Cup	35	5	—	40
Squash, summer variety, hard shell, boiled	1 Cup	90	15	5	110
Tomatoes, canned	1 Cup	40	10	5	55
Tomatoes, raw	1 medium	25	5	5	35
Tomato puŕee, canned	1 Cup	70	20	10	100
Turnips, cooked	1 Cup	35	5	5	45
Turnip greens, boiled	1 Cup	30	15	5	50
Watercress, raw	1 lb.	60	30	10	100

SAT.	UNSAT.	CA.	PHOS.	IRON	SOD.	POT.	A	B₁	B₂	NIA.	C	D
	Fats			*mg.*			*IU*			*mg.*		*IU*
—	—	20	120	1.9	—	200	950	0.3	T	1.7	15	—
—	—	10	25	0.4	T	50	375	T	T	0.4	120	—
—	—	10	50	0.7	5	500	10	T	T	1.2	15	—
—	—	10	50	0.7	5	500	10	T	T	1.2	15	—
—	—	5	30	0.4	700	100	10	T	T	0.6	10	—
H	—	15	75	0.7	5	500	10	T	T	1.8	10	—
H	—	20	90	1.0	10	400	10	T	T	1.5	10	—
—	—	45	150	1.0	600	650	450	0.2	0.1	1.6	15	—
—	—	60	100	1.4	300	10	9000	0.1	T	0.7	25	—
—	—	50	70	1.2	360	15	7000	0.1	0.1	0.6	25	—
—	—	40	85	1.6	5	500	7800	T	0.1	1.2	—	—
—	—	5	50	0.5	5	130	15	T	T	0.1	10	—
—	—	50	20	0.2	15	—	—	T	T	0.3	100	—
—	—	40	20	0.5	800	250	50	T	T	0.1	20	—
—	H	150	350	5.5	5	1000	60	0.4	0.1	1.2	—	—
—	—	20	45	0.7	—	—	150	0.29	0.21	1.0	10	—
—	—	200	70	4.0	600	200	12,000	T	T	0.6	30	—
—	—	10	50	1.0	10	500	700	T	0.1	1.5	10	—
—	—	20	50	1.5	—	500	6000	T	0.1	0.6	10	—
—	—	25	45	1.5	20	550	2500	0.1	T	1.7	40	—
—	—	15	40	0.9	—	300	1500	0.1	T	0.8	35	—
—	—	25	90	2.7	10	400	4500	0.2	0.1	4.5	70	—
—	—	60	50	0.6	10	200	T	T	T	0.4	20	—
—	—	200	70	1.8	75	350	15,000	T	T	0.4	90	—
—	—	20	5	0.2	—	30	400	T	T	0.1	—	—

APPENDIX II
Nutrition-Wise Menu Plans with Between-Meal and Bedtime Snacks

The dietary plans that follow are grouped under three categories —1000, 1600, and 2000 total daily calories. To determine the daily caloric intake and therefore the set of menus appropriate for you, see "Regulate your nutritional intake" in Chapter 5. A snack section follows the menu plans.

NOTE: Dishes with asterisks refer to recipes in Appendix IV.

1000 DAILY CALORIES

Menu 1

BREAKFAST	CARB.	PROT.	FAT	TOTAL
		Cal.		
4 oz. tomato juice, mixed with	20	5	—	25
1½ tsp. brewers' yeast	5	10	—	15
1 egg, soft-poached, topped with	—	25	50	75
2 tsp. vegetable-type bacon	10	60	20	90
1 slice whole-wheat toast	45	10	5	60
Decaffeinated coffee, black	—	—	—	—
	80	110	75	265

MIDMORNING SNACK				
1 peach half, water-pack or unsweetened	15	—	—	15
2 tbsp. cottage cheese, nonfat	5	25	—	30
	20	25	—	45

LUNCH	CARB.	PROT.	FAT	TOTAL
				Cal.
1 chicken fryer thigh, broiled	—	115	35	150
½ Cup green beans	15	—	—	15
3 new potatoes, boiled	45	5	—	50
	60	120	35	215

MIDAFTERNOON SNACK				
1 Cup consomme, plain	—	35	—	35

DINNER				
3 oz. beef tenderloin, grilled	—	130	95	225
Salad plate: place on				
2 lettuce leaves:	5	—	—	5
1 tomato, medium, sliced	25	5	5	35
3 green onions, chopped	10	—	—	10
6 tips asparagus, canned	15	10	5	30
½ tsp. soy oil	—	—	20	20
1 tbsp. vinegar, pure apple	5	—	—	5
Dash of sea salt	—	—	—	—
	60	145	125	330

BEDTIME SNACK				
1 glass (8 oz.) skim milk	50	35	—	85
½ Cup strawberries, fresh or frozen	25	5	—	30
	75	40	—	115

Totals for the day	295	475	235	1005
	(30%)	(47%)	(23%)	

This menu plan provides the following approximate nutrients:

CA.	PHOS.	IRON	SOD.	POT.	A	B₁	B₂	NIA.	C	D
		mg.			IU		mg.			IU
600	1200	15	2000	3000	5500	1.50	2	16	130	30

This menu plan provides the following approximate percent of the Recommended Dietary Allowances:

CA.	PHOS.	IRON	SOD.	POT.	A	B₁	B₂	NIA.	C	D
74%	148%	75%	—	—	111%	150%	122%	129%	232%	—

Menu 2

BREAKFAST	CARB.	PROT.	FAT	TOTAL
		Cal.		
1 orange, sectioned	70	5	5	80
1 egg, scrambled with	—	25	50	75
1½ tsp. brewers' yeast	5	10	—	15
1 pat dietetic margarine	—	—	25	25
1 slice whole-wheat bread	45	10	5	60
Decaffeinated coffee, black	—	—	—	—
	120	50	85	255

MIDMORNING SNACK				
Milk shake: combine in blender				
8 oz. skim milk	50	35	—	85
2 tbsp. wheat germ	15	10	5	30
1½ tsp. brewers' yeast	5	10	—	15
½ medium banana	45	—	—	45
	115	55	5	175

LUNCH				
1 frankfurter, all beef, grilled, topped with	5	60	45	110
½ Cup Sauerkraut	15	5	5	25
1 pear half, water-pack or noncaloric sweetened	15	—	—	15
Dash of ground cloves	—	—	—	—
Tea, hot or cold, noncaloric sweetened	—	—	—	—
	35	65	50	150

MIDAFTERNOON SNACK				
2 tbsp. cottage cheese, nonfat	5	25	—	30
½ Cup celery, raw, diced	10	—	—	10
Dash of cumin	—	—	—	—
	15	25	—	40

DINNER	CARB.	PROT.	FAT	TOTAL
		Cal.		
4 oz. bass, white, steamed,				
garnish with	—	100	15	115
¼ slice lemon	5	—	—	5
1 potato, 2½″ diam., baked	90	10	—	100
1 pat dietetic margarine	—	—	25	25
½ Cup green beans	15	—	—	15
1 slice whole-wheat toast	45	10	5	60
Tea, hot or cold, noncaloric				
sweetened	—	—	—	—
	155	120	45	320

BEDTIME SNACK				
1 Cup consomme, plain, heated	—	35	—	35
1 rye wafer cracker	20	5	—	25
	20	40	—	60

Totals for the day	460	355	185	1000
	(46%)	(35%)	(18%)	

This menu plan provides the following approximate nutrients:

CA.	PHOS.	IRON	SOD.	POT.	A	B₁	B₂	NIA.	C	D
		mg.			*IU*		*mg.*			*IU*
700	1300	15	2300	2500	2600	3.50	3	15	125	55

This menu plan provides the following approximate percent of the Recommended Dietary Allowances:

CA.	PHOS.	IRON	SOD.	POT.	A	B₁	B₂	NIA.	C	D
92%	171%	81%	—	—	53%	350%	185%	122%	232%	—

Menu 3

BREAKFAST	CARB.	PROT.	FAT	TOTAL
			Cal.	
½ Cup salad fruits, water-pack or with				
noncaloric sweetener, topped with	40	—	—	40
2 tbsp. wheat germ	15	10	5	30
1½ oz. dried beef	—	55	25	80
1 egg, soft-poached	—	25	50	75
1 slice whole-wheat bread	45	10	5	60
Decaffeinated coffee, noncaloric				
sweetened	—	—	—	—
	100	100	85	285

MIDMORNING SNACK				
1 peach half, water-pack or noncaloric				
sweetened, topped with	15	—	—	15
2 tbsp. cottage cheese, nonfat	5	25	—	30
Dash of ground cloves	—	—	—	—
	20	25	—	45

LUNCH				
3 oz. liver, beef, broiled with	35	80	55	170
1 tbsp. raw chopped onions	5	—	—	5
½ Cup spinach, cooked	15	10	5	30
½ medium tomato, raw, sliced	10	5	—	15
1 slice whole-wheat bread	45	10	5	60
Tea, hot or cold, noncaloric				
sweetened	—	—	—	—
	110	105	65	280

MIDAFTERNOON SNACK				
1 Cup consomme, hot, plain	—	35	—	35
2 2'' square crackers, saltine-type	20	5	5	30
	20	40	5	65

DINNER	CARB.	PROT.	FAT	TOTAL
		Cal.		
3 oz. chicken livers, boiled	10	75	30	115
½ Cup hominy, cooked	50	5	—	55
½ Cup peas, green	40	15	—	55
1 peach half, water-pack or				
noncaloric sweetened	15	—	—	15
Dash of ground cloves	—	—	—	—
Tea or decaffeinated coffee,				
noncaloric sweetened	—	—	—	—
	115	95	30	240

BEDTIME SNACK				
1 glass (8 oz.) skim milk	50	35	—	85
Totals for the day	415	400	185	1000
	(41%)	(40%)	(19%)	

This menu plan provides the following approximate nutrients:

CA.	PHOS.	IRON	SOD.	POT.	A	B$_1$	B$_2$	NIA.	C	D
		mg.			*IU*		*mg.*			*IU*
675	1850	25	3500	2000	85,500	3.50	8.50	35	100	150

This menu plan provides the following approximate percent of the Recommended Dietary Allowances:

CA.	PHOS.	IRON	SOD.	POT.	A	B$_1$	B$_2$	NIA.	C	D
84%	232%	144%	—	—	1713%	3.80%	565%	256%	186%	—

Menu 4

BREAKFAST	CARB.	PROT.	FAT	TOTAL
		Cal.		
Mix and blend:				
1 glass (8 oz.) skim milk	50	35	—	85
1 tbsp. skim milk powder	15	10	—	25
1½ tsp. brewers' yeast	5	10	—	15
1 egg	—	25	50	75
Noncaloric flavoring to taste	—	—	—	—
1 slice whole-wheat toast	45	10	5	60
1 tbsp. dietetic jelly	—	—	—	—
Decaffeinated coffee, black or noncaloric sweetened	—	—	—	—
	115	90	55	260

MIDMORNING SNACK				
½ Cup strawberries, mixed with	25	5	—	30
4 tbsp. yogurt, nonfat plain	10	5	10	25
	35	10	10	55

LUNCH				
*Baked Tomato with Meat Stuffing	45	40	50	135
6 tips asparagus, steamed	15	10	5	30
½ Cup cabbage, raw, grated	15	—	—	15
½ tsp. soy oil	—	—	20	20
1 tbsp. vinegar, apple cider	5	—	—	5
Dash of sea salt	—	—	—	—
1 slice whole-wheat bread	45	10	5	60
Tea, hot or cold, noncaloric sweetened	—	—	—	—
	125	60	80	265

MIDAFTERNOON SNACK				
1½ oz. tuna, water-pack, on	—	40	25	65
2 2½" square crackers, soda	30	5	10	45
	30	45	35	110

DINNER	CARB.	PROT.	FAT	TOTAL
		Cal.		
3 oz. chipped beef	—	115	50	165
3 new potatoes, boiled	45	5	—	50
Dash of parsley	—	—	—	—
½ Cup spinach, cooked	15	10	5	30
*1 serving Molded Orange Dessert	5	15	—	20
Tea, hot or cold, noncaloric				
sweetened	—	—	—	—
	65	145	55	265

BEDTIME SNACK				
2 peach halves, water-pack or non-				
caloric sweetened, topped with	30	—	—	30
1 tbsp. cottage cheese, nonfat	—	15	—	15
	30	15	—	45

Totals for the day	400	365	235	1000
	(40%)	(37%)	(23%)	

This menu plan provides the following approximate nutrients:

CA.	PHOS.	IRON	SOD.	POT.	A	B₁	B₂	NIA.	C	D
		mg.			*IU*		*mg.*			*IU*
850	1550	20	1700	2800	9800	4	12.5	20	125	40

This menu plan provides the following approximate percent of the Recommended Dietary Allowances:

CA.	PHOS.	IRON	SOD.	POT.	A	B₁	B₂	NIA.	C	D
105%	194%	99%	—	—	195%	397%	840%	165%	224%	—

1600 DAILY CALORIES

Menu 1

BREAKFAST	CARB.	PROT.	FAT	TOTAL
		Cal.		
1 Cup tomato juice, mixed with	45	10	5	60
1½ tsp. brewers' yeast	5	10	—	15
3 oz. beef, lean, ground, broiled	—	90	100	190
1 whole egg plus 1 egg white, scrambled with	—	40	50	90
1 tbsp. skim-milk powder	15	10	—	25
1 slice whole-wheat toast	45	10	5	60
Decaffeinated coffee, black	‒	‒	‒	‒
	110	170	160	440

MIDMORNING SNACK				
½ Cup yogurt, plain, nonfat, topped with	20	15	20	55
½ Cup strawberries, fresh or frozen	25	5	—	30
	45	20	20	85

LUNCH				
*1 serving Curried Beef Pie	25	135	185	345
3 new potatoes, boiled, garnish with	45	5	—	50
Dash of parsley	—	—	—	—
½ medium tomato, raw, sliced	10	5	—	15
1 slice gluten bread	25	30	10	65
1 glass (8 oz.) tea, noncaloric sweetened	‒	‒	‒	‒
	105	175	195	475

MIDAFTERNOON SNACK				
½ Cup cottage cheese, nonfat, mixed with	10	90	5	105
½ Cup celery, raw, diced	10	—	—	10
Dash caraway seeds	‒	‒	‒	‒
	20	90	5	115

DINNER	CARB.	PROT.	FAT	TOTAL
				Cal.
6 oz. shrimp, dry-pack, boiled, topped with	—	180	20	200
*1 serving Seafood Cocktail Sauce	20	—	—	20
*1 serving Carrots and Asparagus au Gratin	20	10	10	40
1 medium young green onion	5	—	—	5
½ tomato, raw, sliced	10	5	—	15
½ medium cucumber, sliced	10	5	—	15
1 slice whole-wheat bread	45	10	5	60
*1 serving Molded Orange Dessert	5	15	—	20
1 glass (8 oz.) tea, noncaloric sweetened	—	—	—	—
	115	225	35	375

BEDTIME SNACK				
1 glass (8 oz.) skim milk, mixed with	50	35	—	85
1 tbsp. skim-milk powder	15	10	—	25
	65	45	—	110
Totals for the day	460	725	415	1600
	(29%)	(45%)	(26%)	

This menu provides the following approximate nutrients:

CA.	PHOS.	IRON	SOD.	POT.	A	B₁	B₂	NIA.	C	D
		mg.			*IU*		*mg.*			*IU*
1350	2000	20	3500	4100	9500	3	23	20	175	75

This menu plan provides the following approximate percent of the Recommended Dietary Allowances:

CA.	PHOS.	IRON	SOD.	POT.	A	B₁	B₂	NIA.	C	D
170%	260%	115%	—	—	190%	300%	1575%	175%	315%	—

Menu 2

BREAKFAST	CARB.	PROT.	FAT	TOTAL
		Cal.		
Milk shake: Combine in blender:				
1 Cup skim milk	50	35	—	85
2 tbsp. skim-milk powder	30	20	—	50
1½ tsp. brewers' yeast	5	10	—	15
½ Cup strawberries, fresh or frozen	25	5	—	30
Non-caloric sweetener to taste	—	—	—	—
3 oz. beef, dried	—	115	50	165
1 slice whole-wheat toast	45	10	5	60
Decaffeinated coffee, black	—	—	—	—
	155	195	55	405

MIDMORNING SNACK				
½ medium (5″ diam.) cantaloupe, filled with	35	5	5	45
2 tbsp. cottage cheese, nonfat	5	25	—	30
	40	30	5	75

LUNCH				
*1 serving Spanish Chicken, served over	30	100	70	200
1 Cup soybean sprouts	25	25	15	65
1 Cup broccoli, seasoned with	35	10	5	50
1 tbsp. lemon juice	5	—	—	5
1 slice gluten bread	25	30	10	65
*1 serving Strawberry Sponge	35	15	—	50
1 glass (8 oz.) tea, noncaloric sweetened	—	—	—	—
	155	180	100	435

MIDAFTERNOON SNACK				
*½ serving Egg Salad with Mushrooms and Cottage Cheese	50	40	30	120
5 small pretzel sticks	10	—	—	10
	60	40	30	130

DINNER	CARB.	PROT.	FAT	TOTAL
		Cal.		
3 oz. beef tenderloin, oven-broiled	—	130	95	225
1 medium potato, baked in jacket, topped with	90	10	—	100
1 pat dietetic margarine	—	—	25	25
1 tbsp. chives	5	—	—	5
½ Cup green beans	15	—	—	15
1 slice whole-wheat bread	45	10	5	60
1 pear half, water-pack or non-caloric sweetened, sprinkled with	15	—	—	15
Dash of ground cloves	—	—	—	—
1 Cup tea, hot, thin slice lemon	5	—	—	5
	175	150	125	450

BEDTIME SNACK				
*1 serving Molded Orange Dessert	5	15	—	20
1 glass (8 oz.) skim milk	50	35	—	85
	55	50	—	105
Totals for the day	640	645	315	1600
	(40%)	(40%)	(20%)	

This menu plan provides the following approximate nutrients:

CA.	PHOS.	IRON	SOD.	POT.	A	B₁	B₂	NIA.	C	D
		mg.			*IU*		*mg.*			*IU*
1400	2400	20	6000	4400	10,500	3	25	45	235	15

This menu plan provides the following approximate percent of the Recommended Dietary Allowances:

CA.	PHOS.	IRON	SOD.	POT.	A	B₁	B₂	NIA.	C	D
175%	300%	115%	—	—	215%	300%	1650%	345%	430%	—

Menu 3

BREAKFAST	CARB.	PROT.	FAT	TOTAL
		Cal.		
1 Cup tomato juice, mixed with	45	10	5	60
1½ tsp. brewers' yeast	5	10	—	15
1 egg, scrambled with	—	25	50	75
3 oz. beef brains	—	35	65	100
1 slice gluten bread, toasted	25	30	10	65
1 tbsp. apple butter, noncaloric				
sweetened	35	—	—	35
Decaffeinated coffee, black	—	—	—	—
	110	110	130	350

MIDMORNING SNACK				
1 all-beef frankfurter, oven-broiled,				
sliced on	5	60	45	110
2 2″ square crackers, saltines	20	5	5	30
1 Cup hot tea, thin slice lemon	5	—	—	5
	30	65	50	145

LUNCH				
½ medium chicken, lean, broiled,				
topped with	—	180	140	320
*1 serving Pimento Cream Sauce	10	5	—	15
½ Cup lima beans	65	20	—	85
1 slice whole-wheat bread	45	10	5	60
1 glass (8 oz.) tea, noncaloric				
sweetened	—	—	—	—
	120	215	145	480

MIDAFTERNOON SNACK				
2 tbsp. skim-milk powder, add				
enough water to whip; place over	30	20	—	50
½ Cup strawberries, fresh or frozen,				
noncaloric sweetened to taste	25	5	—	30
	55	25	—	80

DINNER	CARB.	PROT.	FAT	TOTAL
		Cal.		
4 oz. beef liver, broiled with	40	120	80	240
½ Cup onions, chopped	35	5	5	45
½ Cup spinach, fresh or				
frozen, cooked, topped with	15	10	5	30
2 tsp. vegetable-type bacon	10	60	20	90
1 piece corn bread 2″ x 2″ x ¾″	50	10	20	80
Tea or decaffeinated coffee, non-				
caloric sweetened	—	—	—	—
	150	205	130	485

BEDTIME SNACK				
Combine:				
1 Cup consomme, plain, heated	—	35	—	35
1 envelope unflavored gelatin	—	30	—	30
Dash of celery salt	—	—	—	—
	—	65	—	65

Totals for the day	465	685	455	1605
	(29%)	(43%)	(28%)	

This menu plan provides the following approximate nutrients:

CA.	PHOS.	IRON	SOD.	POT.	A	B₁	B₂	NIA.	C	D
		mg.			*IU*		*mg.*			*IU*
685	2000	25	3100	3200	70,000	3	33	50	170	97

This menu plan provides the following approximate percent of the Recommended Dietary Allowances:

CA.	PHOS.	IRON	SOD.	POT.	A	B₁	B₂	NIA.	C	D
85%	250%	140%	—	—	1400%	300%	2220%	405%	305%	—

Menu 4

BREAKFAST	CARB.	PROT.	FAT	TOTAL
		Cal.		
1 Cup vegetable juice, mixed with	85	5	—	90
1½ tsp. brewers' yeast	5	10	—	15
3 oz. veal cutlet, broiled	—	95	80	175
1 egg, poached	—	25	50	75
1 slice whole-wheat toast	45	10	5	60
Decaffeinated coffee, black	—	—	—	—
	135	145	135	415

MIDMORNING SNACK				
1 pear half, water-pack or non-				
caloric sweetened, topped with	15	—	—	15
2 tbsp. cottage cheese, nonfat	5	25	—	30
1 slice melba toast	30	5	5	40
	50	30	5	85

LUNCH				
4 oz. beef liver, grilled with	40	120	80	240
1 tbsp. raw onions, chopped	5	—	—	5
1 Cup cauliflower, cooked, topped with				
*1 serving Pimento Cream Sauce	10	5	—	15
1 slice whole-wheat bread	45	10	5	60
1 glass (8 oz.) skim milk	50	35	—	85
	175	180	85	440

MIDAFTERNOON SNACK				
1½ oz. dried beef	—	55	25	80
5 small pretzel sticks	10	—	—	10
1 cup tea, hot, thin slice lemon	5	—	—	5
	15	55	25	95

DINNER	CARB.	PROT.	FAT	TOTAL
		Cal.		
3 oz. beef tenderloin	—	130	95	225
1 medium potato, baked, topped with	90	10	—	100
*1 tbsp. Yogurt Herb Dressing	5	5	—	10
Dash of parsley	—	—	—	—
*1 serving Green Bean Salad	35	5	40	80
1 slice gluten bread	25	30	10	65
1 glass (8 oz.) iced tea,				
noncaloric sweetened				
	155	180	145	480

BEDTIME SNACK				
1 glass (8 oz.) buttermilk, nonfat	50	35	—	85
Totals for the day	580	625	395	1600
	(36%)	(39%)	(25%)	

This menu plan provides the following approximate nutrients:

CA.	PHOS.	IRON	SOD.	POT.	A	B₁	B₂	NIA.	C	D
		mg.			*IU*		*mg.*			*IU*
900	2100	25	4000	3700	64,000	2.50	13	28	145	95

This menu plan provides the following approximate percent of the Recommended Dietary Allowances:

CA.	PHOS.	IRON	SOD.	POT.	A	B₁	B₂	NIA.	C	D
113%	268%	148%	—	—	1281%	250%	883%	222%	266%	—

2000 DAILY CALORIES

Menu 1

BREAKFAST	CARB.	PROT.	FAT	TOTAL
		Cal.		
*1 Orange Milk Shake, mixed with	50	25	—	75
1½ tsp. brewers' yeast	5	10	—	15
3 oz. beef tenderloin, oven-broiled	—	130	95	225
1 small biscuit, baking-powder	30	5	10	45
1 tbsp. apple butter	35	—	—	35
	120	170	105	395

MIDMORNING SNACK				
*1 serving Egg Salad with				
Mushrooms and Cottage Cheese	95	75	65	235
1 bouillon cube dissolved in 1 Cup				
of hot water	—	5	—	5
Dash of celery salt	—	—	—	—
	95	80	65	240

LUNCH				
*1 serving Baked Liver Loaf	90	130	95	315
1 Cup spinach, cooked	25	20	10	55
1 medium tomato, raw, sliced	25	5	5	35
1 slice corn bread, 2″ x 2″ x ¾″	50	10	20	80
1 glass (8 oz.) skim milk	50	35	—	85
	240	200	130	570

MIDAFTERNOON SNACK				
1 oz. dry-roasted peanuts	25	30	45	100
1 Cup vegetable juice	85	5	—	90
	110	35	45	190

DINNER	CARB.	PROT.	FAT	TOTAL
		Cal.		
3-oz. beef patty, broiled, served over	—	90	100	190
1 Cup soy sprouts, with	25	25	15	65
*1 tbsp. Vegetable Spaghetti Sauce	25	5	15	45
½ Cup carrots, cooked with	20	—	5	25
½ Cup celery, cooked and	15	—	—	15
1 tbsp. onion, chopped	5	—	—	5
1 slice whole-wheat bread	45	10	5	60
1 glass (8 oz.) tea,				
noncaloric sweetened	=	=	=	=
	135	130	140	405

BEDTIME SNACK				
*1 medium Baked Apple, filled with	80	—	—	80
½ Cup cottage cheese, nonfat, and	10	90	5	105
1½ tsp. brewers' yeast	5	10	=	15
	95	100	5	200

Totals for the day	795	715	490	2000
	(39%)	(36%)	(25%)	

This menu plan provides the following approximate nutrients:

CA.	PHOS.	IRON	SOD.	POT.	A	B_1	B_2	NIA.	C	D
		mg.			*IU*		*mg.*			*IU*
1250	2600	33	4000	4200	33,000	4.5	9	45	215	112

This menu plan provides the following approximate percent of the Recommended Dietary Allowances:

CA.	PHOS.	IRON	SOD.	POT.	A	B_1	B_2	NIA.	C	D
161%	333%	185%	—	—	660%	450%	593%	336%	393%	—

Menu 2

BREAKFAST	CARB.	PROT.	FAT	TOTAL
		Cal.		
½ medium grapefruit, broiled with	100	5	5	110
2 tbsp, wheat germ	15	10	5	30
3 oz. veal cutlet, broiled	—	95	80	175
1 egg, poached, served over	—	25	50	75
1 slice gluten bread	25	30	10	65
Dash of herb seasoning	—	—	—	—
1 glass (8-oz.) skim milk	50	35	—	85
Decaffeinated coffee, black or				
noncaloric sweetened	—	—	—	—
	190	200	150	540
MIDMORNING SNACK				
½ medium cantaloupe, filled with	35	5	5	45
½ Cup cottage cheese, nonfat	10	90	5	105
Dash of nutmeg	—	—	—	—
	45	95	10	150
LUNCH				
*1 serving Baked Liver Loaf	90	130	95	315
1 Cup spinach, fresh, cooked	25	20	10	55
3 medium new potatoes, broiled, topped with	45	5	—	50
Dash of parsley	—	—	—	—
Pat of dietetic margarine and	—	—	25	25
3 young green onions, chopped	10	—	—	10
1 slice whole-wheat bread	45	10	5	60
*1 serving Pineapple Cheese Salad	20	60	—	80
1 glass (8 oz.) tea, noncaloric sweetened				
	225	225	135	595
MIDAFTERNOON SNACK				
1 Cup tomato juice, mixed with	45	10	5	60
1½ tsp. brewers' yeast	5	10	—	15
1 oz. dry-roasted cashews	25	20	50	95
	75	40	55	170

DINNER	CARB.	PROT.	FAT	TOTAL
		Cal.		
*1 serving Spanish Chicken, serve over	30	100	70	200
½ Cup egg noodles	40	5	5	50
Salad:				
1 Cup cabbage, raw, chopped	20	5	—	25
½ Cup celery, raw, diced	10	—	—	10
½ medium green pepper, raw, chopped	10	—	—	10
1 medium carrot, raw, grated	10	—	—	10
1 tsp. vegetable-type bacon	5	30	10	45
2 tbsp. vinegar	10	—	—	10
1 slice melba toast, large	30	5	5	40
Decaffeinated coffee or tea, noncaloric sweetened	—	—	—	—
	165	145	90	400

BEDTIME SNACK				
Combine in blender:				
1 Cup skim milk	50	35	—	85
1 tbsp. skim-milk powder	15	10	—	25
1½ tsp. brewers' yeast	5	10	—	15
1 envelope unflavored gelatin	—	30	—	30
Noncaloric sweetener to taste	—	—	—	—
	70	85	—	155
Totals for the day	770	790	440	2000
	(38%)	(39%)	(23%)	

This menu plan provides the following approximate nutrients:

CA.	PHOS.	IRON	SOD.	POT.	A	B₁	B₂	NIA.	C	D
		mg.			IU		mg.			IU
1750	3500	35	5700	6300	31,500	4.5	20	60	385	130

This menu plan provides the following approximate percent of the Recommended Dietary Allowances:

CA.	PHOS.	IRON	SOD.	POT.	A	B₁	B₂	NIA.	C	D
221%	445%	210%	—	—	632%	450%	1246%	469%	698%	—

Menu 3

BREAKFAST	CARB.	PROT.	FAT	TOTAL
		Cal.		
1 Cup tomato juice, mixed with	45	10	5	60
1½ tsp. brewers' yeast	5	10	—	15
3 oz. beef tenderloin, grilled	—	130	95	225
1 egg, poached	—	25	50	75
1 slice whole-wheat bread	45	10	5	60
Decaffeinated coffee, black	—	—	—	—
	95	185	155	435

MIDMORNING SNACK				
*1 serving Molded Orange Dessert	5	15	—	20
1 glass (8 oz.) skim milk, mixed with	50	35	—	85
1 tbsp. skim-milk powder	15	10	—	25
	70	60	—	130

LUNCH				
*1 serving Curried Beef Pie	25	135	185	345
1 medium baked potato	90	10	—	100
1 Cup string beans	25	5	—	30
1 slice gluten bread	25	30	10	65
*1 medium Baked Apple, topped with	80	—	—	80
2 tbsp. yogurt, nonfat, plain	10	5	—	15
Tea, hot or cold, noncaloric sweetened	—	—	—	—
	255	185	195	635

MIDAFTERNOON SNACK				
1 Cup consomme, plain, serve hot, mixed with	—	35	—	35
1 envelope unflavored gelatin	—	30	—	30
Dash of celery salt	—	—	—	—
1 slice melba toast	30	5	5	40
	30	70	5	105

DINNER	CARB.	PROT.	FAT	TOTAL
		Cal.		
3 oz. veal leg roast	—	110	100	210
1 Cup cauliflower, cooked, topped with	25	10	—	35
*1 tbsp. White Sauce	5	5	5	15
1 ear corn (5″), served with	80	10	5	95
1 pat dietetic margarine and	—	—	25	25
Herb seasoning	—	—	—	—
1 slice gluten bread	25	30	10	65
Tea or decaffeinated coffee, noncaloric sweetened	—	—	—	—
	135	165	145	445

BEDTIME SNACK				
1 Cup cottage cheese, nonfat, mixed with	20	175	10	205
½ Cup blueberries	40	5	—	45
	60	180	10	250

Totals for the day	645	845	510	2000
	(32%)	(42%)	(26%)	

This menu plan provides the following approximate nutrients:

CA.	PHOS.	IRON	SOD.	POT.	A	B$_1$	B$_2$	NIA.	C	D
		mg.			*IU*		*mg.*			*IU*
1150	2400	25	3700	4500	6000	3	12	25	160	40

This menu plan provides the following approximate percent of the Recommended Dietary Allowances:

CA.	PHOS.	IRON	SOD.	POT.	A	B$_1$	B$_2$	NIA.	C	D
145%	300%	145%	—	—	120%	300%	860%	190%	290%	—

Menu 4

BREAKFAST	CARB.	PROT.	FAT	TOTAL
		Cal.		
*1 Baked Apple	80	—	—	80
3 oz. baked ham	—	110	30	140
*1 serving Omelet with Herbs	25	70	100	195
1 slice gluten bread	25	30	10	65
Decaffeinated coffee, black	—	—	—	—
	130	210	140	480

MIDMORNING SNACK				
*1 serving Orange Milk Shake	50	25	—	75
½ Cup yogurt, low-fat, plain	20	15	20	55
	70	40	20	130

LUNCH				
*1 serving Beef Stroganoff	15	110	240	365
½ Cup green peas	40	15	—	55
1 medium ear corn, noncaloric				
seasoning to taste	80	10	5	95
1 slice whole-wheat bread	45	10	5	60
*1 serving Molded Orange Dessert	5	15	—	20
1 Cup hot tea, thin slice lemon	5	—	—	5
	190	160	250	600

MIDAFTERNOON SNACK				
½ Cup cottage cheese, nonfat,	10	90	5	105
on top of				
1 peach half, water-pack or				
noncaloric sweetened	15	—	—	15
Dash of nutmeg	—	—	—	—
	25	90	5	120

DINNER	CARB.	PROT.	FAT	TOTAL
		Cal.		
3 oz. shrimp, fresh, boiled	—	65	5	70
*2 servings Seafood Cocktail Sauce	40	—	—	40
*1 serving Paprika Fish	15	140	40	195
3 new potatoes, boiled, with	45	5	—	50
1 tbsp. onion, raw, chopped	5	—	—	5
*1 serving Carrots and Asparagus				
au Gratin	20	10	10	40
1 slice whole-wheat bread	45	10	5	60
*1 serving Chocolate Fluff	25	20	20	65
1 Cup hot tea, thin slice lemon	5	—	—	5
	200	250	80	530

BEDTIME SNACK				
Combine in blender:				
1 Cup skim milk	50	35	—	85
1 tbsp. skim-milk powder	15	10	—	25
½ Cup strawberries, fresh or frozen	25	5	—	30
	90	50	—	140

Totals for the day	705	800	495	2000
	(35%)	(40%)	(25%)	

This menu plan provides the following approximate nutrients:

CA.	PHOS.	IRON	SOD.	POT.	A	B₁	B₂	NIA.	C	D
		mg.			*IU*		*mg.*			*IU*
1800	3100	25	5000	4700	7200	5	25	30	180	90

This menu plan provides the following approximate percent of the Recommended Dietary Allowances:

CA.	PHOS.	IRON	SOD.	POT.	A	B₁	B₂	NIA.	C	D
225%	395%	135%	—	—	145%	500%	1635%	220%	330%	—

BETWEEN-MEAL AND BEDTIME SNACK SUGGESTIONS

Persons with unstable blood sugar levels require a high protein bedtime and between-meal snack. These combinations will serve as guidelines to supply approximate 200-calorie snacks.

BETWEEN-MEAL SNACKS

CHEESE, EGGS, AND MILK

	MEASURE	CARB.	PROT.	FAT	TOTAL
			Cal.		
Cottage cheese (low-fat)	1 Cup	20	175	10	205
Skim-milk cheese (Edam, Tilsit)	1 oz.	—	40	x60	100
Yogurt (low-fat) plain	½ Cup	20	15	20	55
Hard-boiled eggs	1 medium	—	25	50	75
Buttermilk	1 Cup	50	35	—	85
Skim milk	1 Cup	50	35	—	85

SAT.	UNSAT.	CA.	PHOS.	IRON	SOD.	POT.	A	B₁	B₂	NIA.	C	D
	Fats			*mg.*			*IU*			*mg.*		*IU*
L	L	200	400	0.9	600	180	40	0.1	0.6	0.2	—	—
M	—	210	100	0.1	300	20	350	T	0.1	0.1	—	—
L	L	175	125	T	65	150	75	0.1	0.2	0.1	—	—
H	—	50	200	2.7	80	100	1000	0.1	0.3	0.1	—	30
M	L	120	95	0.1	130	140	T	T	0.2	T	T	T
—	—	305	245	T	150	430	T	0.1	0.5	T	5	T

MEAT, FISH AND POULTRY

	MEASURE	CARB.	PROT.	FAT	TOTAL
			Cal.		
Bacon, vegetable-type	1 tsp.	5	30	10	45
Beef bologna (no additives)	1 slice, 4" x ½" x ⅛"	5	40	50	95
Beef frankfurters (no additives)	1	5	60	45	110
Beef patty (hot)	3 oz.	—	90	100	190
Beef roast, cold	3 oz.	—	80	185	265
Chicken, broiled/boiled	½ lean	—	180	140	320
Chicken livers	3 small, 3 oz.	10	75	30	115
Salmon, canned	3 oz.	—	70	75	145
Sardines, canned in tomato sauce	3 oz.	5	60	115	180
Shrimp, boiled	3 oz.	—	65	5	70
Tuna, water-pack	3 oz.	—	80	50	130
Turkey, roast, cold	3 oz.	—	150	40	190

NUTS AND SEEDS

Almonds, fresh, shelled	10	10	10	x70	90
Cashews, dry-roasted	1 oz.	25	20	50	95
Peanuts, dry-roasted	1 oz.	25	30	45	100
Pumpkin seeds	1 oz.	20	35	115	170
Sunflower seeds	1 oz.	30	25	120	175
Soybeans, roasted or raw	1 oz.	30	55	60	145

SOUPS

Boullion, canned	1 Cup	5	25	—	30
Consomme	1 Cup	—	35	—	35

SAT.	UNSAT.	CA.	PHOS.	IRON	SOD.	POT.	A	B₁	B₂	NIA.	C	D
	Fats			*mg.*			*IU*			*mg.*		*IU*
—	—	—	—	—	—	—	—	—	—	—	—	—
H	L	10	100	2.50	800	200	—	T	T	3.0	—	—
M	L	5	25	.50	400	100	—	0.2	0.2	2.5	—	—
L	L	10	160	3.00	120	350	20	—	—	5.5	—	—
H	L	10	175	3.00	100	350	—	T	0.1	4.5	—	—
L	H	30	420	3.30	175	700	—	0.1	0.3	22.0	—	—
H	L	15	240	7.50	75	300	32,000	0.2	2.5	11.8	20	50
T	H	175	300	1.00	75	300	300	T	0.15	8.5	—	10
L	H	400	200	4.5	400	300	50	T	0.2	5.5	—	50
L	H	100	250	1.5	150	150	20	—	T	2.0	—	10
L	H	10	350	1.4	—	—	20	T	0.1	12.0	—	10
L	H	30	400	5.0	—	—	10	T	0.1	9.0	—	—
T	H	30	70	0.6	T	100	—	T	0.1	0.4	—	—
T	L	15	107	1.0	25	140	—	0.17	0.4	0.7	—	—
M	T	25	135	0.7	T	230	—	0.1	0.4	5.7	—	—
L	H	75	440	8.50	T	—	—	.05	.80	3.40	—	—
L	H	30	200	.50	5	230	—	.90	.10	5.30	—	—
T	T	50	140	1.0	125	275	T	0.33	0.10	0.7	—	—
—	—	—	25	0.2	750	100	—	—	—	0.2	—	—
—	—	—	25	0.2	700	100	—	—	—	0.2	—	—

BEDTIME SNACKS

	MEASURE	CARB.	PROT.	FAT	TOTAL
			Cal.		
Cold roast beef	2 oz.	—	54	122	176
Skimmed milk	1 Cup	50	35	—	85
Total Calories		50	89	122	261
		(19%)	(35%)	(46%)	
Broiled beef patty	2 oz.	—	60	66	126
Hard boiled egg	1	—	25	50	75
Total Calories		—	85	116	201
			(43%)	(57%)	
Water packed tuna	3 oz.	—	80	50	130
Skim milk cheese	1 oz.	—	50	50	100
Total Calories			130	100	230
			(57%)	(43%)	
Chicken livers	3 oz.	10	75	30	115
Skim milk cheese	1 oz.	—	50	50	100
Buttermilk	½ Cup	25	18	—	43
Total Calories		35	143	80	258
		(13%)	(54%)	(33%)	
Hard boiled egg	1	—	25	50	75
Skimmed milk	1 Cup	50	35	—	85
Vegetable type bacon	1 tsp.	5	30	10	45
Total Calories		55	90	60	205
		(26%)	(44%)	(30%)	
All-beef frankfurter	1	5	60	45	110
Skim milk cheese	1 oz.	—	50	50	100
Buttermilk	½ Cup	25	18	—	43
Total Calories		30	128	95	253
		(12%)	(51%)	(37%)	
Boiled shrimp	3 oz.	—	65	5	70
Low fat cottage cheese	½ Cup	10	88	5	103
Buttermilk	½ Cup	25	18	—	43
Total Calories		35	171	10	216
		(16%)	(79%)	(5%)	

SAT.	UNSAT.	CA.	PHOS.	IRON	SOD.	POT.	A	B₁	B₂	NIA.	C	D
Fats				*mg.*			*IU*			*mg.*		*IU*
H	L	7	116	2.0	67	234	—	T	T	3.0	—	—
—	—	305	245	T	150	430	T	.1	.5	T	5	T
L	L	7	106	2.0	80	232	12	T	T	3.6	0	0
H	—	50	200	2.7	80	100	1000	.1	.3	.1	0	30
L	H	10	350	1.4	—	—	20	T	.1	.20	0	0
M	—	210	100	.10	300	20	350	—	.10	.10	—	—
H	L	15	240	7.5	75	300	3200	.2	2.5	11.8	20	50
M	—	210	100	.10	300	20	350	—	.10	.10	—	—
M	L	60	32	T	65	70	T	T	.1	T	T	T
H	—	50	200	2.7	80	100	1000	.1	.3	.1	0	30
—	—	305	245	T	150	420	T	.1	.5	T	5	T
—	—	—	—	—	—	—	—	—	—	—	—	—
M	L	5	25	.5	400	100	—	.2	.2	2.5	—	—
M	—	210	100	.1	300	20	350	—	.1	.1	—	—
M	L	60	32	T	65	70	T	T	.1	T	T	T
L	H	100	250	1.5	150	150	20	—	T	2.0	—	10
L	L	100	200	T	300	90	20	.5	.3	.1	—	—
M	L	60	32	T	65	70	T	T	.1	T	T	T

BEDTIME SNACKS (continued)

	MEASURE	CARB.	PROT.	FAT	TOTAL
			Cal.		
Boiled shrimp	3 oz.	—	65	5	70
Boiled egg	1	—	25	50	75
Skimmed milk	½ Cup	25	18	—	43
Total Calories		25	108	55	188
		(12%)	(58%)	(40%)	
Roasted turkey	2 oz.	—	100	27	127
Skim milk cheese	1 oz.	—	50	50	100
Total Calories		—	150	77	227
			(70%)	(30%)	
Chicken thigh					
(broiled, skin removed)	1 med.	—	115	35	150
Skimmed milk	½ Cup	25	18	—	43
Total Calories		25	133	35	193
		(13%)	(69%)	(18%)	
Broiled beef patty	2 oz.	—	60	66	126
Cottage cheese (low fat),					
mixed in with the patty	4 tbsp.	—	40	—	40
Total Calories		—	100	66	166
			(60%)	(40%)	
Dried beef	3 oz.	—	115	50	165
Low fat cottage cheese	2 tbsp.	—	20	—	20
Total Calories		—	135	50	185
			(74%)	(26%)	
Water pack tuna	2 oz.	—	53	33	86
Boiled egg	1	—	25	50	75
Bouillon	1 Cup	—	5	—	5
Total Calories		—	83	83	166
			(50%)	(50%)	
Low fat cottage					
cheese, sprinkle with,	½ Cup	10	88	5	103
Vegetable type bacon	2 tsp.	10	60	20	90
Total Calories		20	148	25	193
		(12%)	(75%)	(13%)	

SAT.	UNSAT.	CA.	PHOS.	IRON	SOD.	POT.	A	B₁	B₂	NIA.	C	D
Fats				*mg.*			*IU*			*mg.*		*IU*
L	H	100	250	1.5	150	150	20	—	T	2.0	—	10
H	—	50	200	2.7	80	100	1000	.1	.3	.1	—	30
—	—	153	123	T	75	215	T	.1	.5	T	3	T
L	H	20	134	3.4	—	—	7	T	T	6.0	—	—
M	—	210	100	.1	300	20	350	—	.1	.1	—	—
L	M	15	200	1.0	100	300	—	.1	.1	8.0	—	—
—	—	153	123	T	75	215	T	.1	.5	T	3	T
L	L	7	106	2.0	80	232	12	T	T	3.6	—	—
L	L	50	100	T	150	44	10	T	T	T	—	—
L	L	15	300	1.5	3000	150	—	T	.2	3.0	—	—
L	L	50	50	T	75	22	5	T	T	T	—	—
L	H	7	232	1.0	—	—	12	T	T	8.0	—	7
H	—	50	200	2.7	80	100	1000	.1	.3	.1	—	30
—	—	—	—	.1	100	10	—	—	—	—	—	—
L	L	100	200	T	300	90	20	.5	.3	.1	—	—
—	—	—	—	—	—	—	—	—	—	—	—	—

BEDTIME SNACKS (continued)

	MEASURE	CARB.	PROT.	FAT	TOTAL
			Cal.		
Broiled beef patty	2 oz.	—	60	66	126
Skim milk cheese	1 oz.	—	50	50	100
Total Calories		—	110	116	226
			(49%)	(51%)	
Canned salmon	3 oz.	—	70	50	120
Skimmed milk	1 Cup	50	35	—	85
Total Calories		50	105	50	205
		(24%)	(52%)	(24%)	
Water pack tuna	3 oz.	—	80	50	130
Boiled egg	1	—	25	50	75
Total Calories		—	105	100	205
			(52%)	(48%)	
All beef bologna	1 slice	5	40	50	95
Skim milk cheese	1 oz.	—	50	50	100
Total Calories		5	90	100	195
		(2%)	(46%)	(52%)	
Chicken livers	3 oz.	10	75	30	115
Buttermilk	1 Cup	50	35	—	85
Total Calories		60	105	30	195
		(30%)	(54%)	(16%)	
Canned sardines, natural pack	3 oz.	5	60	115	180
Skimmed milk	½ Cup	25	18	—	43
Total Calories		30	78	115	223
		(14%)	(35%)	(49%)	

SAT.	UNSAT.	CA.	PHOS.	IRON	SOD.	POT.	A	B$_1$	B$_2$	NIA.	C	D
Fats				*mg.*			*IU*			*mg.*		*IU*
L	L	7	106	2.0	80	232	12	T	T	3.6	—	—
M	—	210	100	.1	300	20	350	—	.1	.1	—	—
T	H	175	300	1.0	75	300	100	T	.1	8.5	—	—
—	—	305	245	T	150	420	T	.1	.5	T	5	T
L	H	10	350	1.4	—	—	20	T	.1	.2	—	—
H	—	50	200	2.7	80	100	1000	.1	.3	.1	—	30
H	L	10	100	2.5	800	200	—	—	—	3.0	—	—
M	—	210	100	.1	300	20	350	—	.1	.1	—	—
H	L	15	240	7.5	75	300	3200	.2	2.5	11.8	20	50
M	L	120	95	.1	130	140	T	T	.2	T	T	T
L	H	400	200	4.5	400	300	50	—	.2	5.5	—	50
—	—	153	123	T	75	215	T	.1	.5	T	3	T

APPENDIX III
Converting Your Favorite Recipes

To convert your favorite recipes to ones that are nutrition-wise, follow these step-by-step instructions:

  A. List the amounts of all of the ingredients in the recipe.
  B. Look up the number of calories of fats, protein, and carbohydrates, as well as the total calories of each ingredient, in Appendix I.
  C. Write down these caloric valuations of fat, protein, and carbohydrates and also the total caloric estimation in their respective columns.
  D. Total all columns of figures for the entire recipe.
  E. Divide the totals of each column by the number of individual servings in the recipe to determine the caloric amounts of fats, protein, and carbohydrates as well as the total calories in each individual serving.
  F. Study the nutrition-wise recipes in Appendix IV and the Refrigerator Cheesecake recipes that follow to get accustomed to the substitute ingredients used (for example, yogurt or blended cottage cheese for sour cream; wheat germ for bread crumbs) and also refer to nutrition-wise boosters listed in Chapter 5.
  G. After making as many substitutions as you can, refer again to the nutrition-wise boosters listed in Chapter 5 and try to include one or more of these ingredients to further enhance and augment the nutritional values of your modified recipe.

REGULAR RECIPE

REFRIGERATOR CHEESECAKE	CARB.	PROT.	FAT	TOTAL
		Cal.		
3 tbsp. butter, softened	—	—	300	300
1 Cup graham cracker crumbs	200	30	50	280
2 envelopes unflavored gelatin	—	60	—	60
¾ Cup cold water	—	—	—	—
2 egg yolks, beaten	—	20	100	120
¾ Cup milk	40	30	65	135
½ Cup sugar	385	—	—	385
¼ tsp. salt	—	—	—	—
1 8-oz. package cream cheese	15	80	760	855
1 tsp. lemon rind, grated	5	—	—	5
1 tsp. vanilla extract	10	—	—	10
2 tbsp. sugar	100	—	—	100
1 tbsp. lemon juice	5	—	—	5
2 egg whites, stiffly beaten	—	30	—	30
1¼ Cup whipping cream	—	—	1000	1000
Totals in 10 servings:	760	250	2275	3285
Totals in 1 serving:	75	25	225	325
	(23%)	(8%)	(69%)	

1. Make the crust with the softened butter and graham cracker crumbs. Press into 8-inch springform pan. Bake in preheated oven at 400° for 10 minutes. Cool while preparing the filling.
2. Soften the gelatin in ¾ cup cold water in top of double boiler. Let stand for 5 minutes.
3. To the gelatin mixture, add the beaten egg yolks, milk, sugar, salt, and cream cheese. Cook over low heat, stirring constantly, until mixture slightly thickens.
4. Add lemon rind, vanilla, 2 tbsp. sugar, and lemon juice. Remove from heat to cool.
5. Beat the egg whites and whipping cream separately. Fold both into the cheese mixture. Pour into crust and chill until set.

NUTRITIONAL ANALYSIS OF
REFRIGERATOR CHEESECAKE

REGULAR RECIPE

This recipe provides the following approximate nutrients in 10 servings:

CA.	PHOS.	IRON	SOD.	POT.	A	B$_1$	B$_2$	NIA.	C	D
		mg.			IU		mg.			IU
660	1785	9.45	3120	1005	9690	1.65	6.15	1.70	16.25	250

This recipe provides the following approximate nutrients in 1 serving:

CA.	PHOS.	IRON	SOD.	POT.	A	B$_1$	B$_2$	NIA.	C	D
		mg.			IU		mg.			IU
65	180	0.95	310	100	970	0.15	0.60	0.15	1.6	25

NUTRITION-WISE CONVERTED RECIPE

REFRIGERATOR CHEESECAKE	CARB.	PROT.	FAT	TOTAL
		Cal.		
2 tbsps. butter or margarine	—	—	200	200
½ Cup graham cracker crumbs (5 crackers)	100	15	25	140
¼ Cup wheat germ	35	20	10	65
¾ Cup skim milk	40	25	—	65
½ Cup nonfat dry milk solids	75	50	—	125
3 Cups cottage cheese, low-fat	60	525	30	615
2 envelopes unflavored gelatin	—	60	—	60
¾ Cup cold water	—	—	—	—
2 egg yolks	—	20	100	120
2 tbsps. sugar	100	—	—	100
2 tbsps. liquid noncaloric sweetener	—	—	—	—
1 tbsp. lemon juice	5	—	—	5
¼ tsp. sea salt	—	—	—	—
1 tsp. grated lemon rind	5	—	—	5
1 tsp. vanilla extract	10	—	—	10
2 egg whites, stiffly beaten	—	30	—	30
Totals in 10 servings:	430	745	365	1550
Totals in 1 serving:	40	75	35	155
	(28%)	(48%)	(24%)	

1. Soften butter. Add cracker crumbs and wheat germ. Press firmly into bottom and sides of 8-inch springform pan. Bake in preheated hot oven (400°) for 10 minutes. Cool.
2. Combine skim milk, nonfat dry milk solids, and cottage cheese in blender.
3. Soften the gelatin in ¾ cup cold water in top of double boiler. Let stand for 5 minutes.
4. To the gelatin mixture beat in the egg yolks and sugar and cook, stirring constantly, until slightly thickened. Add blended cottage cheese and milk, noncaloric sweetener, and flavorings to the hot mixture.
5. Carefully fold the hot mixture into the beaten egg whites. Pour into prepared crumb crust and chill until firm.

NUTRITIONAL ANALYSIS OF
REFRIGERATOR CHEESECAKE

NUTRITION-WISE CONVERTED RECIPE

This recipe provides the following approximate nutrients in 10 servings:

CA.	PHOS.	IRON mg.	SOD.	POT.	A IU	B₁	B₂ mg.	NIA.	C	D IU
1535	2555	11.75	3100	1020	1260	1.3	86.25	3.05	20	110

This recipe provides the following approximate nutrients in 1 serving:

CA.	PHOS.	IRON mg.	SOD.	POT.	A IU	B₁	B₂ mg.	NIA.	C	D IU
153	255	1.17	310	102	126	0.13	8.62	0.3	2	11

APPENDIX IV
NUTRITION-WISE RECIPES

BEVERAGES

Orange Milk Shake

1 Cup skim milk
½ Cup orange juice,
   fresh or unsweetened
1 egg white, stiffly beaten
1 tsp. orange peel, grated
½ Cup cracked ice

1. Place milk, orange juice, orange peel, and ice in an electric blender or shaker. Mix or shake until blended in.
2. Add the egg white and mix only until well blended.

	CARB.	PROT.	FAT	TOTAL
		Cal.		
Total caloric values—2 servings	100	55	—	155
Values in 1 Portion—1 serving	50	25	—	75
Percent of caloric values	67%	33%	—	

This recipe provides the following approximate nutrients:

CA.	PHOS.	IRON	SOD.	POT.	A	B$_1$	B$_2$	NIA.	C	D
		mg.			*IU*		*mg.*			*IU*
175	140	0.3	95	345	115	0.05	0.3	0.1	33	—

This recipe provides the following approximate percent of the Recommended Dietary Allowances:

CA.	PHOS.	IRON	SOD.	POT.	A	B$_1$	B$_2$	NIA.	C	D
22%	17%	1%	—	—	2%	5%	22%	1%	59%	—

DESSERTS

Baked Apple

1 medium apple
⅛ tsp. cinnamon
⅛ tsp. ground cloves
1 tbsp. water
Noncaloric sweetener to taste

1. Wash and core apple.
2. Place in shallow baking dish.
3. Mix spices and water together; pour over apple.
4. Bake in moderate (350°F.) oven until done, about 35 minutes.

	CARB.	PROT.	FAT	TOTAL
		Cal.		
Total caloric value—1 serving	80	—	—	80
Percent of caloric values	100%	—	—	

This recipe provides the following approximate nutrients:

CA.	PHOS.	IRON	SOD.	POT.	A	B₁	B₂	NIA.	C	D
		mg.			IU		mg.			IU
5	10	0.3	—	75	100	—	—	0.2	15	—

This recipe provides the following approximate percent of the Recommended Dietary Allowances:

CA.	PHOS.	IRON	SOD.	POT.	A	B₁	B₂	NIA.	C	D
1%	1%	2%	—	—	2%	—	—	2%	27%	—

Chocolate Fluff

1 envelope unflavored gelatin
2 Cups skim milk
1 square unsweetened chocolate
⅜ tsp. liquid noncaloric sweetener
¼ tsp. vanilla
⅛ tsp. cinnamon

1. Soften gelatin in the milk in the top of a double boiler. Add the chocolate and cinnamon. Heat over boiling water, stirring constantly until the chocolate and gelatin dissolve. Remove from heat.
2. Add the noncaloric sweetener and vanilla.
3. Chill until mixture is the consistency of unbeaten egg whites.
4. Set pan in ice water and beat until mixture becomes double in volume.
5. Spoon into 6 individual custard cups. Chill until firm.

	CARB.	PROT.	FAT	TOTAL
		Cal.		
Total caloric values—6 servings	135	105	135	375
Values in 1 portion—1 serving	25	20	20	65
Percent of caloric values	38%	31%	31%	

This recipe provides the following approximate nutrients:

CA.	PHOS.	IRON	SOD.	POT.	A	B₁	B₂	NIA.	C	D
		mg.			IU		mg.			IU
105	95	0.3	50	155	T	T	0.17	0.03	2	—

This recipe provides the following approximate percent of the Recommended Dietary Allowances:

CA.	PHOS.	IRON	SOD.	POT.	A	B₁	B₂	NIA.	C	D
13%	12%	2%	—	—	—	3%	11%	—	3%	—

Molded Orange Dessert

1 envelope unflavored gelatin
2 tbsps. orange juice
1 Cup boiling water
½ tsp. liquid noncaloric sweetener
Rind of ½ orange, grated

1. Soften the gelatin in the orange juice. Dissolve in the boiling water.
2. Add the noncaloric sweetener and the grated orange rind. Pour into individual molds and chill until firm.

	CARB.	PROT.	FAT	TOTAL
		Cal.		
Total caloric values—2 servings	10	30	—	40
Values in 1 portion—1 serving	5	15	—	20
Percent of caloric values	25%	75%	—	

This recipe provides the following approximate nutrients:

CA.	PHOS.	IRON	SOD.	POT.	A	B$_1$	B$_2$	NIA.	C	D
		mg.			*IU*		*mg.*			*IU*
5	5	0.1	T	30	30	—	—	T	5	—

This recipe provides the following approximate percent of the Recommended Dietary Allowances:

CA.	PHOS.	IRON	SOD.	POT.	A	B$_1$	B$_2$	NIA.	C	D
1%	—	—	—	—	1%	—	—	—	14%	—

Strawberry Sponge

2 Cups fresh strawberries, washed and drained
1 envelope unflavored gelatin
Hot water
1 Cup orange juice, fresh or unsweetened
1½ tbsp. liquid noncaloric sweetener
2 egg whites, stiffly beaten
⅛ tsp. almond extract
Dash of salt, sea or vegetable

1. Reserve 6 strawberries to use for garnish. Force the remaining berries through a food mill or mash them.
2. Soften the gelatin in the orange juice. Place over hot water and stir until dissolved. Add the noncaloric sweetener. Cool until the mixture begins to thicken.
3. Add the berries, and beat until the mixture is foamy. Fold in the egg whites, almond extract and salt.
4. Arrange the 6 whole strawberries on the bottom of a 1-quart mold. Pour the sponge mixture all over them and chill until set.

	CARB.	PROT.	FAT	TOTAL
		Cal.		
Total caloric values–6 servings	205	80	15	300
Values in 1 portion–1 serving	35	15	—	50
Percent of caloric values	70%	30%		

This recipe provides the following approximate nutrients:

CA.	PHOS.	IRON	SOD.	POT.	A	B₁	B₂	NIA.	C	D
	mg.				*IU*		*mg.*			*IU*
30	25	T	35	185	110	—	0.1	0.2	55	—

This recipe provides the following approximate percent of the Recommended Dietary Allowances:

CA.	PHOS.	IRON	SOD.	POT.	A	B₁	B₂	NIA.	C	D
4%	3%	3%	—	—	2%	—	3%	2%	97%	—

EGGS

Omelet with Herbs

4 eggs
2 tbsp. skim-milk powder
½ tsp. sea salt
1 tbsp. mixture of dry herbs:
   tarragon, chervil, basil, and chives
¼ Cup skim milk
1½ tsp. brewers' yeast
Dash of pure ground black pepper

1. Separate egg yolks and whites.
2. Beat egg whites until stiff but not dry.
3. Beat egg yolks until thick and lemon-colored.
4. Add salt, herb mixture, milk, brewers' yeast, and pepper.
5. Fold the egg yolk mixture into the whites.
6. Pour into a hot, lightly buttered omelet pan or skillet. Cook over low heat until omelet has risen and is golden brown next to pan. Then set the pan in a preheated moderate oven for 5 minutes, or until surface seems set.
7. Serve at once, piping hot.

	CARB.	PROT.	FAT	TOTAL
		Cal.		
Total caloric values—2 servings	50	140	200	390
Values in 1 portion—1 serving	25	70	100	195
Percent of caloric values	13%	36%	51%	

This recipe provides the following approximate nutrients:

CA.	PHOS.	IRON	SOD.	POT.	A	B_1	B_2	NIA.	C	D
		mg.			IU		mg.			IU
225	525	5	770	305	2005	0.6	10	1	T	60

This recipe provides the following approximate percent of the Recommended Dietary Allowances:

CA.	PHOS.	IRON	SOD.	POT.	A	B_1	B_2	NIA.	C	D
9%	38%	23%	—	—	34%	15%	30%	1%	—	—

FISH AND SEAFOOD

Paprika Fish

1 tbsp. butter or margarine
2 tsp. paprika
2 tsp. salt, sea or vegetable
½ tsp. pepper
1 Cup onions, chopped
2 lbs. white fish
1 Cup water
½ Cup yogurt, plain

1. Melt the butter or margarine in a heavy skillet. Saute the onions until lightly browned. Stir in the paprika.
2. Arrange the fish over the onions, add the salt and pepper, and put in the water. Bring to a boil.
3. Cover and cook over low heat 45 minutes.
4. Remove the fish to a serving dish. Stir the yogurt into the sauce and heat, but do not boil. Pour over the fish and serve.

	CARB.	PROT.	FAT	TOTAL
		Cal.		
Total caloric values—6 servings	100	835	225	1160
Values in 1 portion—1 serving	15	140	40	195
Percent of caloric values	8%	72%	20%	

This recipe provides the following approximate nutrients:

CA.	PHOS.	IRON	SOD.	POT.	A	B$_1$	B$_2$	NIA.	C	D
		mg.			*IU*		*mg.*			*IU*
175	495	T	895	630	115	0.2	0.2	5	5	20

This recipe provides the following approximate percent of the Recommended Dietary Allowances:

CA.	PHOS.	IRON	SOD.	POT.	A	B$_1$	B$_2$	NIA.	C	D
22%	62%	14%	—	—	2%	20%	15%	58%	6%	—

MEAT

Baked Liver Loaf

1 lb. beef liver
½ Cup soft bread crumbs (whole wheat)
½ Cup wheat germ
1 egg, slightly beaten
1 tsp. salt, sea or vegetable
¼ Cup onion, chopped
1 Cup skim milk

1. Place liver into boiling salted water and cook 5 to 10 minutes.
2. Grind liver and onion in a food chopper.
3. Mix together the bread crumbs, wheat germ, egg, milk, and salt. Stir in the ground liver and onion and mix well.
4. Put into a baking dish and set into a pan of hot water. Bake at 350°F. for 30 minutes.

	CARB.	PROT.	FAT	TOTAL
		Cal.		
Total caloric values—4 servings	360	525	375	1260
Values in 1 portion—1 serving	90	130	95	315
Percent of caloric values	29%	41%	30%	

This recipe provides the following approximate nutrients:

CA.	PHOS.	IRON	SOD.	POT.	A	B₁	B₂	NIA.	C	D
		mg.			IU		mg.			IU
130	735	10	840	620	7240	0.5	4	20	45	80

This recipe provides the following approximate percent of the Recommended Dietary Allowances:

CA.	PHOS.	IRON	SOD.	POT.	A	B₁	B₂	NIA.	C	D
17%	91%	63%	—	—	145%	54%	325%	155%	80%	—

Baked Tomato with Meat Stuffing

4 medium tomatoes
Salt and pepper
1 tsp. butter or margarine
2 tbsp. onion, chopped
¼ lb. ground round beef
¼ Cup soft bread crumbs
¼ Cup wheat germ
⅛ tsp. basil
¼ tsp. salt, sea or vegetable
¼ tsp. Worchestershire sauce
2 tbsp. cold water

1. Remove tops from tomatoes and scoop out the pulp. Salt and pepper the inside of the tomatoes.
2. Melt the butter or margarine in a small skillet. Saute the onion until lightly browned. Add meat and cook over low heat until the meat is browned.
3. Remove meat from the heat and stir in the bread crumbs and wheat germ. Add the remaining ingredients. Mix well.
4. Fill tomatoes with the meat mixture. Place in a shallow baking dish and add ¼ cup hot water.
5. Bake at 375°F. for 25 minutes.

	CARB.	PROT.	FAT	TOTAL
		Cal.		
Total caloric values—4 servings	170	165	205	540
Values in 1 portion—1 serving	45	40	50	135
Percent of caloric values	33%	30%	37%	

This recipe provides the following approximate nutrients:

CA.	PHOS.	IRON	SOD.	POT.	A	B₁	B₂	NIA.	C	D
		mg.			*IU*		*mg.*			*IU*
35	175	5	215	430	1560	0.2	0.1	5	35	5

This recipe provides the following approximate percent of the Recommended Dietary Allowances:

CA.	PHOS.	IRON	SOD.	POT.	A	B₁	B₂	NIA.	C	D
4%	22%	16%	—	—	31%	21%	8%	24%	64%	—

Beef Stroganoff

2 lb. sirloin steak, ¼-inch thick
3 tbsp. onion, grated
1 tbsp. butter or margarine
1-1½ Cups mushrooms, sliced
¼ tsp. basil
1 tsp. salt
½ tsp. pepper
6 tbsp. yogurt

1. Trim all excess fat from the meat. Pound meat with a mallet and cut into strips.
2. In a skillet, saute the onion in the melted butter until lightly browned. Add the steak strips and continue browning.
3. Remove the beef. Saute the mushrooms; return the beef to the skillet and season with the basil, salt, and pepper.
4. Add the yogurt; heat but do not let boil.

	CARB.	PROT.	FAT	TOTAL
		Cal.		
Total caloric values—8 servings	100	890	1935	2925
Values in 1 portion—1 serving	15	110	240	365
Percent of caloric values	4%	30%	66%	

This recipe provides the following approximate nutrients:

CA.	PHOS.	IRON	SOD.	POT.	A	B₁	B₂	NIA.	C	D
	mg.				IU		mg.			IU
35	250	5	360	515	100	0.01	0.1	5	T	T

This recipe provides the following approximate percent of the Recommended Dietary Allowances:

CA.	PHOS.	IRON	SOD.	POT.	A	B₁	B₂	NIA.	C	D
4%	31%	21%	—	—	2%	1%	9%	51%	2%	—

Curried Beef Pie

½ Cup onions, chopped
1 tsp. butter or margarine
1 slice whole-wheat bread, crumbled
½ Cup skim milk
1¼ lb. ground round beef
2 eggs
1 tbsp. curry powder
1 tbsp. lemon juice
1 tsp. salt, sea or vegetable
2 tbsp. ground almonds

1. In a heavy saucepan or skillet, saute the onion in the melted butter or margarine.
2. Soak the bread in the milk. Drain. Mix thoroughly the bread, beef, onions, 1 egg, curry powder, lemon juice, salt, and almonds.
3. Spoon the meat mixture into a 9-inch pie pan.
4. Beat the remaining egg with the milk in which the bread was soaked. Pour over the meat.
5. Bake for 1 hour in a 350°F. oven.

	CARB.	PROT.	FAT	TOTAL
		Cal.		
Total caloric values—6 servings	140	815	1115	2070
Values in 1 portion—1 serving	25	134	185	345
Percent of caloric values	7%	39%	54%	

This recipe provides the following approximate nutrients:

CA.	PHOS.	IRON	SOD.	POT.	A	B$_1$	B$_2$	NIA.	C	D
		mg.			IU		mg.			IU
75	310	5	615	540	380	0.2	0.2	10	10	10

This recipe provides the following approximate percent of the Recommended Dietary Allowances:

CA.	PHOS.	IRON	SOD.	POT.	A	B$_1$	B$_2$	NIA.	C	D
9%	39%	26%	—	—	8%	26%	19%	52%	13%	—

Spanish Chicken

1 2-lb. broiler, disjointed
1 medium green pepper, chopped
½ Cup capers
1 tsp. salt, sea or vegetable
2 tomatoes, chopped
¼ Cup onion, chopped
20 large green olives, chopped
1 small pimento, chopped

1. Remove the skin and excess fat from the chicken.
2. Place all ingredients in a heavy saucepan. Cover with water.
3. Cover and simmer 1½ hours, or until the chicken falls from the bone.
4. Remove bones and serve.

	CARB.	PROT.	FAT	TOTAL
		Cal.		
Total caloric values—4 servings	125	405	270	800
Values in 1 portion—1 serving	30	100	70	200
Percent of caloric values	15%	50%	35%	

This recipe provides the following approximate nutrients:

CA.	PHOS.	IRON	SOD.	POT.	A	B_1	B_2	NIA.	C	D
	mg.				IU		mg.			IU
60	295	3	1160	530	1070	0.1	0.2	10	35	—

This recipe provides the following approximate percent of the Recommended Dietary Allowances:

CA.	PHOS.	IRON	SOD.	POT.	A	B_1	B_2	NIA.	C	D
7%	37%	17%	—	—	21%	18%	17%	84%	61%	—

SALADS AND SPREADS

Egg Salad with Mushrooms and Cottage Cheese

4 eggs, hard-cooked
½ Cup cottage cheese, low-fat
¼ Cup mushrooms, sliced
1 tsp. Worcestershire sauce
1 tsp. lemon juice
1 tsp. celery seeds
*2 tbsp. Special Mayonnaise
 Salt, pepper, and paprika to taste

1. Finely chop or mash the hard-cooked eggs. Blend cottage cheese to the consistency of cream cheese. Add eggs to cheese.
2. Stir in the mushrooms, Worcestershire sauce, lemon juice, celery seeds, and Special Mayonnaise.
3. Season to taste.

	CARB.	PROT.	FAT	TOTAL
		Cal.		
Total caloric values—4 servings	385	280	255	920
Values in 1 portion—1 serving	95	75	65	235
Percent of caloric values	40%	32%	28%	

This recipe provides the following approximate nutrients:

CA.	PHOS.	IRON	SOD.	POT.	A	B₁	B₂	NIA.	C	D
		mg.			IU		mg.			IU
77	260	5	225	140	1005	0.1	0.4	0.5	5	T

This recipe provides the following approximate percent of the Recommended Dietary Allowances:

CA.	PHOS.	IRON	SOD.	POT.	A	B₁	B₂	NIA.	C	D
10%	32%	16%	—	—	20%	11%	27%	4%	5%	—

Green Bean Salad

2 tbsp. vegetable salad oil
3 medium onions, chopped
4 Cups fresh or frozen (thawed) green
   beans
1 Cup tomato juice
1 tsp. salt, sea or vegetable
½ tsp. black pepper

1. In a saucepan, heat the oil and saute
   the onions until brown.
2. Add the beans, tomato juice, salt, and pepper.
3. Cover and cook over low heat 25 minutes.

	CARB.	PROT.	FAT	TOTAL
		Cal.		
Total caloric values—6 servings	215	30	255	500
Values in 1 portion—1 serving	35	5	40	80
Percent of caloric values	44%	6%	50%	

This recipe provides the following approximate nutrients:

CA.	PHOS.	IRON	SOD.	POT.	A	B₁	B₂	NIA.	C	D
		mg.			IU		mg.			IU
35	25	0.5	495	215	850	—	—	0.5	10	—

This recipe provides the following approximate percent of the Recommended Dietary Allowances:

CA.	PHOS.	IRON	SOD.	POT.	A	B₁	B₂	NIA.	C	D
4%	3%	3%	—	—	17%	—	—	3%	14%	—

Pineapple-Cheese Salad

½ envelope unflavored gelatin
¼ Cup cold water
¼ Cup hot water
½ tsp. vinegar
1 tbsp. lemon juice
¼ tsp. sea salt
4 tbsp. cottage cheese
2 tbsp. crushed pineapple, water-pack
   or noncaloric sweetened
Lettuce leaf
Noncaloric sweetener to taste

1. Soften the gelatin in the cold water. Dissolve in the hot water. Add the vinegar, lemon juice, and salt.
2. Chill until of the consistency of unbeaten egg whites.
3. Fold in the cottage cheese and pineapple. Chill until firm. Pour into an individual mold.
4. Unmold and serve on lettuce leaf.

	CARB.	PROT.	FAT	TOTAL
		Cal.		
Total caloric value—1 serving	20	60	—	80
Percent of caloric values	25%	75%	—	

This recipe provides the following approximate nutrients:

CA.	PHOS.	IRON	SOD.	POT.	A	B₁	B₂	NIA.	C	D
		mg.			IU		mg.			IU
110	130	T	740	320	1020	0.1	0.1	0.5	60	—

This recipe provides the following approximate percent of the Recommended Dietary Allowances:

CA.	PHOS.	IRON	SOD.	POT.	A	B₁	B₂	NIA.	C	D
14%	16%	7%	—	—	20%	13%	10%	3%	109%	—

Vitamin Spread

1 Cup carrots, grated
½ medium green pepper
3 stalks celery
2 tbsp. wheat germ
2 tbsp. walnuts, chopped
1 tbsp. prepared horseradish
*3 tbsp. Special Mayonnaise
1 tsp. lemon juice
Salt, sea or vegetable, to taste

1. Grind together the three vegetables.
2. Add the wheat germ, walnuts, horseradish, Special Mayonnaise, and lemon juice. Season to taste with the salt.
3. Serve on low-calorie crackers, toasted whole-wheat bread rounds, or melba toast, or stuff celery sticks.

	CARB.	PROT.	FAT	TOTAL
		Cal.		
Total caloric values—2 Cups	110	45	115	270
Values in 1 portion—1 tbsp.	5	5	—	10
Percent of caloric values	50%	50%	—	

This recipe provides the following approximate nutrients:

CA.	PHOS.	IRON	SOD.	POT.	A	B₁	B₂	NIA.	C	D
		mg.			IU		mg.			IU
5	15	0.15	20	15	105	T	T	0.1	5	T

This recipe provides the following approximate percent of the Recommended Dietary Allowances:

CA.	PHOS.	IRON	SOD.	POT.	A	B₁	B₂	NIA.	C	D
1%	2%	1%	—	—	2%	1%	1%	1%	9%	—

SAUCES AND DRESSINGS

Pimento Cream Sauce

5 tbsp. nonfat dry milk solids
1 tsp. cornstarch
½ Cup lukewarm water
1 bouillon cube
1 canned pimento, slivered
Salt, sea or vegetable, and pepper

1. In a small saucepan, blend together the milk solids and cornstarch. Add the water and stir until smooth.
2. Add the bouillon cube. Bring the mixture to a boil, stirring constantly.
3. Lower heat and add the pimento. Simmer until all ingredients are well blended.
4. Season to taste with the salt and pepper.

	CARB.	PROT.	FAT	TOTAL
		Cal.		
Total caloric values—½ Cup	90	30	—	120
Values in 1 portion—1 tbsp.	10	5	—	15
Percent of caloric values	67%	33%		

This recipe provides the following approximate nutrients:

CA.	PHOS.	IRON	SOD.	POT.	A	B$_1$	B$_2$	NIA.	C	D
		mg.			IU		mg.			IU
50	35	0.2	20	10	305	T	10	T	T	—

This recipe provides the following approximate percent of the Recommended Dietary Allowances:

CA.	PHOS.	IRON	SOD.	POT.	A	B$_1$	B$_2$	NIA.	C	D
6%	4%	2%	—	—	6%	1%	413%	—	1%	—

Seafood Cocktail Sauce

Pinch of salt, sea or vegetable
2 tbsp. malt vinegar
¼ tsp. Worcestershire sauce
¼ tsp. Tabasco sauce
3 tbsp. catsup
2 tbsp. horseradish, grated
3 tbsp. chili sauce

1. Add the salt to the vinegar, and stir in the Worcestershire sauce.
2. Mix in the Tabasco, catsup, horseradish, and chili sauce. Blend.

	CARB.	PROT.	FAT	TOTAL
		Cal.		
Total caloric values—6 servings	125	—	—	125
Values in 1 portion—1 serving	20	—	—	20
Percent of caloric values	100%			

This recipe provides the following approximate nutrients:

CA.	PHOS.	IRON	SOD.	POT.	A	B₁	B₂	NIA.	C	D
		mg.			*IU*		*mg.*			*IU*
5	5	0.1	125	50	300	—	—	—	—	—

This recipe provides the following approximate percent of the Recommended Dietary Allowances:

CA.	PHOS.	IRON	SOD.	POT.	A	B₁	B₂	NIA.	C	D
—	1%	1%	—	—	6%	—	—	—	—	—

White Sauce

1 tbsp. flour
½ Cup nonfat dry milk solids
½ tsp. sea salt
⅛ tsp. white pepper
1 Cup water
1 tbsp. dietetic margarine

1. In a saucepan, mix the flour, dry milk, salt, and pepper.
2. Add the water and beat until smooth.
3. Cook over low heat, stirring constantly until the sauce thickens.
4. Stir in the butter or margarine. Sauce will be thin.

	CARB.	PROT.	FAT	TOTAL
		Cal.		
Total caloric values—1 Cup	95	50	100	245
Values in 1 portion—1 tbsp.	5	5	5	15
Percent of caloric values	33%	33%	33%	

This recipe provides the following approximate nutrients:

CA.	PHOS.	IRON	SOD.	POT.	A	B₁	B₂	NIA.	C	D
	mg.				*IU*		*mg.*			*IU*
40	30	T	80	10	30	T	5	T	30	—

This recipe provides the following approximate percent of the Recommended Dietary Allowances:

CA.	PHOS.	IRON	SOD.	POT.	A	B₁	B₂	NIA.	C	D
5%	4%	—	—	—	1%	1%	333%	—	1%	—

Yogurt Herb Dressing

3 tbsp. lemon juice
1 tsp. salt, sea or vegetable
¼ tsp. prepared mustard
1 Cup yogurt, plain

1. Mix lemon juice and salt, blending in mustard.
2. Gradually add to the yogurt, blending thoroughly.
3. Chill for at least ½ hour before using.

	CARB.	PROT.	FAT	TOTAL
		Cal.		
Total caloric values—20 tbsp.	90	70	60	220
Values in 1 portion—1 tbsp.	5	5	—	10
Percent of caloric values	50%	50%	—	

This recipe provides the following approximate nutrients:

CA.	PHOS.	IRON	SOD.	POT.	A	B₁	B₂	NIA.	C	D
	mg.				IU		mg.			IU
20	15	—	125	15	10	T	T	T	5	—

This recipe provides the following approximate percent of the Recommended Dietary Allowances:

CA.	PHOS.	IRON	SOD.	POT.	A	B₁	B₂	NIA.	C	D
2%	2%	—	—	—	—	1%	1%	—	8%	—

Vegetable Spaghetti Sauce

1 bouillon cube
1½ Cup boiling water
¼ clove of garlic
Dash of sea salt
1 tsp. butter or margarine
4 large mushrooms, sliced (about 1
    Cup)
1 green pepper, minced
¼ onion, minced
½ tomato, cubed
Dash dry mustard
Paprika to taste

1. Dissolve the bouillon cube in boiling water.
2. Rub the saucepan with the garlic and salt. Melt the butter or margarine.
3. Saute the mushrooms, green pepper, and onion until brown.
4. Add the bouillon liquid and tomato. Cover and simmer for 15 minutes.
   Season to taste with the dry mustard and paprika.

	CARB.	PROT.	FAT	TOTAL
		Cal.		
Total caloric values—3 servings	80	20	40	140
Values in 1 portion—1 serving	25	5	15	45
Percent of caloric values	56%	11%	33%	

This recipe provides the following approximate nutrients.

CA.	PHOS.	IRON	SOD.	POT.	A	B_1	B_2	NIA.	C	D
		mg.			*IU*		*mg.*			*IU*
15	70	.5	290	210	395	T	.2	5	45	T

This recipe provides the following approximate percent of the Recommended Dietary Allowances:

CA.	PHOS.	IRON	SOD.	POT.	A	B_1	B_2	NIA.	C	D
2%	9%	4%	—	—	8%	2%	13%	17%	77%	—

Special Mayonnaise

1 cup yogurt, plain
1 hard-cooked egg, finely chopped
1 tbsp. lemon juice
¼ tsp. celery seed or curry
¼ tsp. prepared mustard
½ tsp. salt, sea or vegetable

1. Mix all ingredients thoroughly.
2. Chill for at least ½ hour before using.

	CARB.	PROT.	FAT	TOTAL
		Cal.		
Total caloric values—1 Cup	85	95	110	290
Values in 1 portion—1 tbsp.	5	5	5	15
Percent of caloric values	33%	33%	33%	

This recipe provides the following approximate nutrients:

CA.	PHOS.	IRON	SOD.	POT.	A	B₁	B₂	NIA.	C	D
	mg.				*IU*		*mg.*			*IU*
25	28.44	0.17	86	25	71.88	0.02	0.04	0.02	1.88	2

This recipe provides the following approximate percent of the Recommended Dietary Allowances:

CA.	PHOS.	IRON	SOD.	POT.	A	B₁	B₂	NIA.	C	D
3%	4%	1%	—	—	1%	2%	3%	—	3%	—

VEGETABLES

Carrots and Asparagus au Gratin

1½ Cups carrots, cooked, diced
1½ tbsp. chopped parsley
12 stalks asparagus, cooked
½ Cup bouillon (made with a cube)
2 tbsp. dry cheddar cheese, grated

1. Mix together the carrots, parsley, and asparagus. Place in a shallow baking dish.
2. Pour bouillon over the vegetables and sprinkle with the cheese.
3. Bake, uncovered, in a 350°F. oven, 20 to 25 minutes.

	CARB.	PROT.	FAT	TOTAL
		Cal.		
Total caloric values—4 servings	80	35	35	150
Values in 1 portion—1 serving	20	10	10	40
Percent of caloric values	50%	25%	25%	

This recipe provides the following approximate nutrients:

CA.	PHOS.	IRON	SOD.	POT.	A	B₁	B₂	NIA.	C	D
		mg.			IU		mg.			IU
60	60	T	255	115	3460	T	0.1	1	10	—

This recipe provides the following approximate percent of the Recommended Dietary Allowances:

CA.	PHOS.	IRON	SOD.	POT.	A	B₁	B₂	NIA.	C	D
7%	8%	6%	—	—	69%	5%	7%	7%	14%	—

Index